Mammography, Thermography and Ultrasonography in Breast Disease

Kenneth T. Evans
M.B., Ch.B., D.M.R.D., F.R.C.P., F.F.R.
Professor of Diagnostic Radiology, Welsh National School of Medicine; Director, Department of Diagnostic Radiology, University Hospital of Wales

and

I. Huw Gravelle
B.Sc., M.B., Ch.B., D.M.R.D., F.R.C.P., F.F.R.
Consultant Radiologist, University Hospital of Wales; Clinical Teacher in Diagnostic Radiology, Welsh National School of Medicine

Butterworths

ENGLAND: BUTTERWORTH & CO. (PUBLISHERS) LTD.
                   LONDON: 88 Kingsway, WC2B 6AB

AUSTRALIA: BUTTERWORTHS PTY. LTD.
                   SYDNEY: 586 Pacific Highway, 2067
                   MELBOURNE: 343 Little Collins Street, 3000
                   BRISBANE: 240 Queen Street, 4000

CANADA: BUTTERWORTH & CO. (CANADA) LTD.
                   TORONTO: 14 Curity Avenue, 374

NEW ZEALAND: BUTTERWORTHS OF NEW ZEALAND LTD.
                   WELLINGTON: 26–28 Waring Taylor Street, 1

SOUTH AFRICA: BUTTERWORTH & CO. (SOUTH AFRICA) (PTY.) LTD.
                   DURBAN: 152–154 Gale Street

Suggested U.D.C. Number: 618·19–073

ISBN 0 407 26450 7

Made and printed in Great Britain by
William Clowes & Sons, Limited, London, Beccles and Colchester

Contents

Editor's Foreword

In the seventy-five years or so of its life diagnostic radiology has grown from a scientific toy into a useful tool and from an occasional luxury into a diagnostic necessity. Today it performs an important role in clinical diagnosis. Radiologists are no longer isolated from their colleagues in dark basements. They now form an integral part of the team, comprising many specialties, whose object is successful patient management. Collaboration and mutual understanding between the various members and some appreciation of the value and limitations of their several disciplines is obviously necessary.

It is to this end that this book has been written and forms part of the series Radiology in Clinical Diagnosis. The purpose of the series is to give clinicians an up-to-date and comprehensive survey of the role of diagnostic radiology in different spheres of clinical practice and to provide radiologists in training with a hand-book from which they can quickly learn and to which they can readily refer. The books have been written, illustrated and printed so that they will be comprehensive without being exhaustive. We very much hope they will prove a pleasure for the individual to own and to use as well as a standard text for the library shelf.

Much has been written on mammography and there are numerous papers describing thermography of the breast. On the other hand, ultrasonic examination of the breast requires such specialized equipment that it has not been so widely used or described.

These different methods of investigating breast disease and the principles on which each depends are brought together, clearly and helpfully described and evaluated in this monograph. The superiority of mammography over the other methods of examination is well shown. However the complementary role of the various techniques is also demonstrated.

For the Clinician and the Radiologist here is a splendid collection of illustrations which should provide a concise and yet comprehensive guide to imaging techniques in breast disease.

Westminster Hospital, London   DAVID H. TRAPNELL

Preface

Sophisticated methods have been developed in recent years for the investigation of patients with breast disease. In this book we have attempted to evaluate the place of mammography, thermography and ultrasound.

We have discussed the interpretation of mammograms according to the presenting radiographic abnormality and not according to clinical or histological criteria. We believe that this will be a more useful method of presentation.

Thermography is not yet wholly evaluated as a technique in the assessment of breast disease and we present our experience of this method fully realizing that our conclusions will not be accepted by some other workers.

Our experience of ultrasound in the investigation of breast disease is limited but we feel that it may develop as an important additional physical method of investigation.

It gives us great pleasure to acknowledge the help we have received from the Surgeons in Cardiff particularly those from the Surgical Unit, formerly under the directorship of Professor A. P. M. Forrest, and now under Professor L. E. Hughes.

We are indebted to Dr. J. N. Wolfe for kindly allowing us to reproduce the xeroradiographs in *Figure 1.3*. Our thanks are also due to Professor P. N. T. Wells for the development of our ultrasonic apparatus and for help in numerous ways. From Professor Wells' book *Physical Principles of Ultrasonic Diagnosis*, published by Academic Press, we reproduce *Figures 5.5, 5.7* and *5.9* and we are grateful for permission to make use of these sonograms.

We wish to thank Aga (UK) Limited for permission to use the schematic illustration of the Aga Thermovision in *Figure 4.1* and the Editor of *X-ray Focus*, published by Ilford Limited, for permission to include a number of illustrations in Chapter 2.

We are particularly grateful to the Tenovus Organisation for financial assistance in purchasing the Aga Thermovision, for our ultrasonic apparatus and for assisting us in the development of our mammography service over the years.

Reproduction of mammograms is particularly difficult and we wish to acknowledge the enormous help we have received from Mr. R. J. Marshall and his staff in the Department of Medical Illustration and also from Mrs. P. Ware and Mrs. J. Cooke in the Department of Illustration of the Dental School.

Again, we are indebted to the many Radiographers who have assisted us with our projects in mammography, thermography and ultrasonography; their co-operation has been invaluable.

Finally, our sincere thanks are due to Mrs. R. E. Moss for her diligence and secretarial expertise during the preparation of this monograph.

Cardiff   KENNETH T. EVANS
                                                        I. HUW GRAVELLE

Chapter 1

Techniques of Mammography

HISTORY

Radiography was first employed in the investigation of breast cancer by Salomon in 1913. He correlated the radiographic features of operative specimens with their pathological features and the results of direct examination.

In 1930, Warren described a radiographic study of the breast and Gershon-Cohen's original paper on the early diagnosis of mammary cancer by means of mammography appeared in 1937. Hicken (1937) also published a paper on mammography in that year advocating the use of contrast media. He produced excellent radiographs depicting normal and abnormal lactiferous ducts, cysts, papillomas and carcinomas. He recommended the use of Thorotrast, being unaware of its potential dangers.

Since 1937 Gershon-Cohen has published many important papers on mammography and together with Ingleby (1960) he has placed this technique on a sound anatomical and pathological basis.

The credit for the development and perfection of a reliable and reproducible mammographic technique goes to Leborgne (1953). His recognition and description of numerous characteristic radiological stages must be acknowledged.

In more recent years soft tissue radiographic techniques of breast examination have become generally accepted and excellent reviews have been published by Gros (1963), Egan (1964; 1970) and Samuel and Young (1964).

Mammography is the technique of examination of the breast by means of low energy radiography. This may be carried out by conventional mammography, 70 mm photofluorography, fluidography and xeroradiography. Additional information may be obtained by enhancing the low natural contrast of the breast by use of a positive

1

contrast medium to outline the ducts and a double contrast technique to outline cysts.

The term 'conventional mammography' is used to denote the process by which full sized radiographs of the breasts are obtained without the use of contrast media and without immersion of the breasts in liquid. The comments on technique which follow apply to conventional mammography, positive contrast examination of the ducts and double contrast examination of cysts. Variations used in fluidography, xerography and 70 mm photofluorography will be mentioned separately.

TECHNIQUES OF EXAMINATION

Apparatus

Several commercial units are now available which have been specifically designed for mammography. Each has its individual features but in general all units are constructed to operate at a low kilovoltage and with fine focal spots. The target metal is either tungsten or molybdenum with or without a rotating anode. In some, inherent tube filtration only is used and in others beryllium windows with added low filtration.

In conventional x-ray tubes the x-ray beam consists of radiation of varying wavelengths. The radiation of long wavelengths is readily absorbed by the glass tube envelope and by added filters, usually of aluminium. It is these low energy x-rays that are needed for the production of soft tissue radiographs as in mammography. Consequently it is necessary to preserve these rays by reducing the inherent filtration of the glass envelope and discarding the usual added aluminium filters. In some types of apparatus a beryllium window is used in the tube to reduce the filtration further. However, in such apparatus added filtration is essential to avoid skin damage by low energy x-rays.

Units have been designed so that the tube can rotate, allowing both supero-inferior and medio-lateral projections to be taken with the patient remaining in the erect position. Even though this facility reduces the examination time it is more difficult to project the retromammary fat and chest wall on to the films in the medio-lateral position.

It is not proposed to discuss the merits and demerits of the various sophisticated mammographic systems now commercially available. It is sufficient to state that excellent results are obtainable with all these units. Equally good results can also be achieved using inexpensive conversions of standard radiographic equipment. The unit used in our Department consists of a modified Watson Roentgen IV generator allowing normal radiography on the overcouch tube up to

2

90 kVp and restricting output for mammography from approximately 20 kVp to 40 kVp.

This generator is used in conjunction with a Machlett Dynamax HD 40 tube designed for mammography. It has a twin filament assembly placed nearer the target than in standard tubes and the primary beam exit in the glass insert is ground down. This reduces inherent filtration which is equivalent to approximately 0·4 mm aluminium. There is a rotating tungsten anode and the foci measure 1 mm and 2 mm. With added filtration this can be used for conventional overcouch radiography. The 2 mm focus is used for mammography at a 300 mA setting and although there is a theoretical possibility of filament overheating at low voltages the tube has been in constant use for mammography and standard radiography for 7 years.

To enable thorough examination of the mammograms to be made, special viewing arrangements must be available. The Picker High Intensity Illuminator Model 185 and the 'Mavig' Mammoscop provide the appropriate illumination for such examination.

Radiographic Projections

In every examination at least two views of each breast are essential and these should be taken at right-angles to each other so that a non-palpable pathological process can be accurately localized to a quadrant of the breast. In conjunction with the basic supero-inferior and medio-lateral projections, an 'axillary tail' view in the supero-inferior position ensures that the whole of the breast is visualized in the horizontal plane. If any doubt remains as to the character of a lesion a localized radiograph is taken in an appropriate position.

Occasionally an axillary view is taken when there is some doubt as to whether or not there are enlarged axillary nodes present. This projection shows the contents of the axilla and also provides another view of the axillary tail of the breast. Lymph nodes are frequently shown but it should be appreciated that nodes of normal size may contain metastases and enlargement may not be the result of malignant deposits.

In our technique one lead marker is placed over a palpable lesion, two over apparently normal breasts and three over the scar of a previous biopsy. This is helpful in subsequent interpretation of the mammograms and may be seen in many of the illustrations.

These lead markers can be attached to the breast with Sellotape but care should be taken that the skin is not wrinkled by the tape because this may give the misleading appearance of localized skin thickening.

3

Films of 24 × 18 cm size are adequate. It is usually possible to take a supero-inferior view on one half of a 24 × 18 cm film and the axillary tail view on the other half. A whole film is used for every medio-lateral projection so that a portion of the chest wall may be included. A whole 24 × 18 cm film is needed for the axillary projection and for a supero-inferior view of large breasts.

Film markers and patient identification numbers are combined and are routinely placed on the lateral aspect of the breast in the supero-inferior views and on the superior aspect of the breast in the medio-lateral projections. This facilitates rapid orientation during viewing of the mammograms.

Supero-inferior Projection

An adjustable stand is used for this position—the patient standing

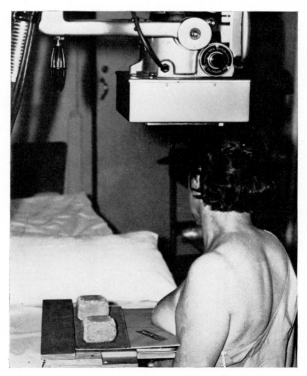

Figure 1.1. Position for the supero-inferior projection. The film is on an Iontomat plate and centering is to the base of the breast with the nipple in profile

4

or being seated on a stool close to this. An Iontomat plate containing a special mammography chamber is placed on the stand so that the chamber will eventually be situated beneath the thickest part of the breast—that is, towards the base. The film is then placed on the Iontomat plate and the breast positioned on the film. The stand is adjusted so as to be as comfortable as possible for the patient. The film is placed against the chest wall and the under-surface of the breast should be in contact with the film and free of skin wrinkles. In addition the nipple should be in profile (*Figure 1.1*).

The patient's head is turned away from the breast being examined and the shoulder on that side allowed to drop backwards. This helps to eliminate the shadow caused by the clavicle. The unused half of the film is covered by lead rubber and the x-ray beam is collimated to within a few millimetres of the breast. A portion of the chest wall should be included but the whole of the retro-mammary fat area is not usually seen in this projection. The beam is directed to the middle of the base of the breast.

Axillary Tail Projection

Because the axillary tail of the breast is not often completely visualized on the conventional supero-inferior view it is advisable to include this on the remaining half of the supero-inferior film. The position is virtually the same as that used for the supero-inferior projection but the Iontomat plate and film are moved laterally and the patient turns medially so that the Iontomat plate and film lie underneath the axillary tail region. Collimation of the beam includes the axillary tail, the lateral half of the breast and a little of the chest wall. The central ray is directed to the base of the breast.

Medio-lateral Projection

For this projection (*Figure 1.2*) it is best to have the patient in the recumbent position as the retro-mammary fat space can then be demonstrated in all cases. When this projection is taken with the patient in the erect position it is not always possible to show the retro-mammary space adequately.

The patient first lies supine on the x-ray table and then turns towards the side being examined. At this stage the film is placed in direct contact with the breast and inserted so that it lies under and in contact with the chest wall. It is helpful to bend the film gently before placing it in position so that its convex side can be moulded to the chest wall and lateral aspect of the breast. Blocks of wood approximately half an inch thick are now inserted beneath the film to support it. The Iontomat plate is inserted on top of the wooden blocks

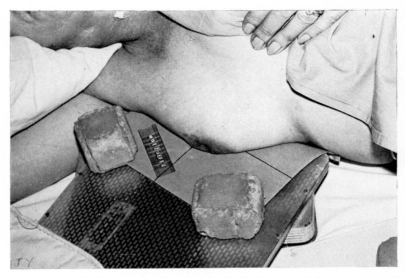

Figure 1.2. Medio-lateral view. Note how the film is closely applied to the chest and the Iontomat plate is elevated on wooden blocks

and directly beneath the film with the chamber under the base of the breast. Finally the patient is rotated on to the film so that the nipple is in profile. The opposite breast is drawn back by the patient. It may be necessary to support the patient in this position by means of pillows and sandbags. The x-ray beam is accurately collimated and approximately an inch and a half of chest wall is included on the film. The beam is centred to the middle of the base of the breast.

Axillary Projection

The axillary view is also best carried out in the recumbent position. The Iontomat plate and film are placed lengthwise under the axilla and the patient turned 25–30 degrees towards the axilla. The arm is abducted to 90 degrees and the beam centred a few centimetres below the apex of the axilla. The breast is not in direct contact with the film in this position but useful views of the axillary tail of the breast may be obtained.

Technical Factors

The normal structures of the breast and often the pathological lesions within the breast consist of tissues which exhibit little difference in their propensity for absorbing radiation. Consequently to

6

produce a satisfactory diagnostic mammogram it is necessary to apply the principles of soft tissue radiography.

A low kilovoltage, a high milliamperage and a relatively prolonged exposure time are required. Blurring is minimized by the use of a fine focus, a short object–film distance and an anode–film distance of not less than 76 cm. Compression of the breast and support of the patient will reduce loss of sharpness due to movement. With low energy radiation a low filtration of the beam is necessary and collimation is important. The use of fine grain, non-screen film and subsequent hand processing of the film complete the requirements for soft tissue radiography.

Theoretically all these principles should be applied but in practice it is usually necessary to achieve a compromise between the various factors.

Kilovoltage

A low kilovoltage of the order of 20–35 kV is necessary. The kilovoltage used will vary with the projection and the type of film and of breast being radiographed. An immature glandular breast or a lactating breast will need a higher kV than an atrophic fatty breast. In addition, the thickness of the base of the breast should be taken into consideration but only after the breast has been positioned accurately. The factors used in our Department are shown in Table 1.1.

TABLE 1.1

Projection	kVp*	Type of film
Supero-inferior and axillary tail	21–27	Industrex C (Kodak Ltd.)
Medio-lateral	18–21	Osray M film (Agfa Gevaert)
Axillary view	31	Osray M film (Agfa Gevaert)

* With compression a reduction of 3 kVp can be achieved.

Individual x-ray units will vary so that it is advisable to make test exposures using a step wedge and phantom until radiographs of satisfactory quality are produced.

Milliamperage

With the low kilovoltage a high enough milliamperage to give good contrast is essential. Our unit has a fixed setting of 300 mA which is used for all projections. At the low kilovoltages used the effective milliamperage will be less—due to the space charge effect. The true reading on our unit is about 280 mA.

Exposure Time

A relatively long exposure time is required and it is advisable but not essential to employ some automatic method of exposure control. We use an Iontomat with a chamber specially produced for mammography; a photo-timer would do equally well. The exact time is not known but is of the order of 3 seconds for the supero-inferior and axillary tail projections using industrial film, 2·5 seconds for the medio-lateral view using medical non-screen film and approximately 3 seconds for the axillary projection which is taken on medical non-screen film also.

The Geometrics of the Radiographic System

Theoretically a fine focal spot is advantageous for obtaining detail and fine resolution. It is obligatory if a short target film distance is used. However with techniques using a high mAs value a fine focal spot cannot be used. In practice there is little loss of detail on films using a 2 mm focus at an anode film distance of 76 cm and an mA setting of 300.

The object–film distance should be as short as possible and in practice the breast is in direct contact with the double wrapped film.

Filtration and Collimation

As previously explained the use of a low kilovoltage necessitates low filtration of the x-ray beam so that there is minimal absorption of the low energy radiation and consequent enhancement of contrast. No additional filtration is used on our unit. That obtained is the inherent filtration of the tube itself (equivalent to 0·4 mm of aluminium).

Collimation of the x-ray beam reduces scatter and so increases contrast. Many authorities advocate the use of copper or lead lined cones of varying lengths but these are not essential. Indeed it is frequently difficult using cones to include a portion of the chest wall on the film. A specially modified light beam diaphragm can be used but it is necessary to replace the standard reflecting mirror by a thin silvered perspex mirror which has a negligible filtration value. Collimation with a light beam diaphragm is rapid and accurate and a portion of the chest wall can be easily included on the film. The retro-mammary fat space is then well demonstrated on all medio-lateral projections.

Compression and Reduction of Movement

It is possible to compress the breast by a compression device made of a low absorption material such as expanded polystyrene which is usually incorporated in the end of an extension cone. It is not necessary to use compression routinely but if the breast consists of dense glandular or fibrous tissue gentle compression is employed by means of a polystyrene plate. The plate is placed directly on the breast and kept in position by lead weights. Compression of the breast is also valuable to reduce movement in nervous patients.

As the exposure time is relatively long there is a likelihood of movement blurring. Movement can be minimized by reassuring a nervous patient and explaining the procedure beforehand. If the patient is kept comfortable by the use of pillows and sandbags and encouraged to relax it will reduce the possibility of motion blurring due to patient movement and forceful heart action. The exposure is made during arrested respiration.

Film and Processing

As many of the breast structures are extremely fine and microcalcification characteristic of malignancy is often minute in size, non-screen, fine grain film is required for the detailed demonstration of breast architecture and pathology. There are two main schools of thought regarding the type of film used in mammography (Egan, 1970; Gershon-Cohen et al., 1965). It is argued by Egan on the one hand that a fine grain industrial type of film is required in order to show in detail the normal architecture of the breast and the pathological processes. He maintains that it is more important to reduce motion than to reduce the long exposure time. Gershon-Cohen on the other hand maintains that the increased contrast obtained by using medical non-screen film and a relatively short exposure time is more advantageous and that microcalcification is more easily shown in this way.

This argument can be resolved by using a combination of these techniques. An industrial type film (Industrex C—Kodak Ltd.) can be used for the supero-inferior and axillary tail views and the medio-lateral and axillary views can be taken on medical non-screen film (Osray M—Agfa Gevaert). In this way mammograms of different quality are obtained of each breast and so a more comprehensive examination is effected.

Medichrome, a blue-based film produced by Agfa Gevaert Ltd., can be used for mammography. By viewing the mammogram through a series of filters different structures and tissues are brought into prominence. It is doubtful whether this film has any advantages over conventional film. No cases have been reported of malignant lesions shown on Medichrome film that were not visible on conventional black and white film.

A further modification that has been reported (Price and Butler, 1970) is the use of industrial type film and medical non-screen film with a back mounted, high definition, tungstate intensifying screen. The film is vacuum packed in an Amplatz vacuum cassette. Using this system excellent mammograms can be obtained with reduction in exposure time.

Hand processing is recommended for the films mentioned above. Industrial film has a thick emulsion and so requires a development time of 10 minutes. The medical non-screen film is developed for 5 minutes. Both are processed in a low energy developer at a temperature of 68°F (20°C). After rinsing, fixation takes 15 minutes and the films are then washed in running water for 20–25 minutes. They may then be dried in a drying cabinet or rapid drying unit.

It is now possible to obtain film (PE 4006—Kodak Ltd.; Type S film—3M Company) comparable to industrial type that can be rapidly processed in 90 seconds in an automatic processor.

Table 1.2 summarizes the technical factors used by the authors and compares these factors with those used by Egan and Gershon-Cohen.

The skin radiation dosages obtained using these techniques are 4 rads for the supero-inferior projection and axillary tail view and 3 rads for the medio-lateral view using the Cardiff method. Gershon-Cohen states that his technique gives about 1 rad in both the supero-inferior and medio-lateral projection (Gershon-Cohen et al., 1965). Egan maintains that with his method of examination the dosages are 2·4 rads for the supero-inferior view and 2·8 rads for the medio-lateral view. The dosage for the axillary view is not stated (Egan, 1968). However, Gilbertson et al. (1970) report that the skin doses using Egan's technique are much higher than this and may reach a maximum of 18 R when all three views are taken.

Mammograms of excellent quality can be obtained using the technical details outlined above but in some instances additional information can be obtained by contrast examinations.

POSITIVE CONTRAST EXAMINATION OF THE DUCTS

Positive contrast examination of the duct system of the breast is a rapid, safe and painless procedure (Hicken, 1937; Leborgne, 1953; Bjørn-Hansen, 1965). Its main use is in the investigation of nipple discharge but it can also be used to differentiate between benign and malignant masses in the breast. A benign lesion may displace a duct without infiltration but a malignant lesion may cause an irregular filling defect or stricture.

10

TABLE 1.2

	Egan	*Gershon-Cohen*	*Cardiff*
Routine projections	Supero–inferior (S.i.) Medio–lateral (M.l.) Axillary	Supero-inferior Medio-lateral	Supero-inferior Axillary tail Medio–lateral (axillary)
kVp	20–30 S.i. and M.l. 54 axillary	25–32 S.i. and M.l.	18–27 (31 axillary)
mA	300 (approx: 240–260)	mAs 200–400	300 (approx: 280)
Exposure time	6 sec—S.i. view 6 sec—M.l. view 3·5 sec—axillary		Iontomat S.i. about 3 sec Axillary tail— about 3 sec M.l. about 2·5 sec Axillary about 2·5 sec.
Anode-film distance (AFD)	S.i. and M.l. 56–102 cm Axillary 76–102 cm	S.i. and M.l. 36 cm	4 views—76 cm
Focal spot	2·0 mm	0·8 mm	2·0 mm
Filtration	Inherent tube filtration only	Inherent tube filtration only	Inherent tube filtration only
Collimation	Cones	Cones	Modified light beam diaphragm
Compression	None	Cone compression	Occasional with polystyrene plate
Film	Industrial film for 3 views	Medical non-screen film for both views	Industrial film for S.i. and axillary tail view Medical non-screen film for M.l. and axillary view

Routine mammograms are first obtained. Cannulation of the duct is initially carried out in the supine position and the patient then rotated into the position for the medio-lateral view. The procedure is then repeated with the patient erect and positioned for the supero-inferior view.

The nipple and areola are cleaned with spirit and the discharging duct orifice demonstrated following gentle pressure on all quadrants of the breast in turn. If the problem is one of differentiation of a mass and there is no discharge the appropriate quadrant of the nipple is selected following clinical examination of the breast and scrutiny of the preliminary mammograms. In such cases the duct orifices may be difficult to locate. This task is made easier by first smearing the nipple with a little olive oil and then mopping up the excess oil with a swab. The positions of the duct orifices are then visible because droplets of the oil will tend to remain in the ostia. The use of magnifying spectacles will facilitate this procedure.

Following selection of the appropriate duct orifice gentle dilatation is carried out using a graduated series of lachrymal probes. Usually a lachrymal cannula can then be inserted easily into the duct. Before insertion of the cannula it is vital to ensure that there is no air in the injection system. Immediately prior to injection the patient is positioned for the medio-lateral view. Contrast medium (25 per cent Hypaque) is then injected slowly and without force until the patient experiences a feeling of fullness in the breast. When this occurs the injection is stopped and the exposure made with the cannula in position. The procedure is repeated with the patient positioned for the cranio-caudal view when the cannula usually slips easily into the duct without prior probing of the duct orifice. The volume of medium usually required is 0·5–2·0 ml for each injection. When the ducts are very large a greater volume will be required and this may be judged approximately from the preliminary mammograms. The exact volume required will be determined by the response of the patient. At the end of the examination the medium is expressed. No complications of this procedure have been encountered.

DOUBLE CONTRAST EXAMINATION OF CYSTS

A double contrast method may be used to outline cysts. This has the advantage of showing the inner walls of cystic lesions. The skin overlying the cyst is infiltrated with a small amount of a local anaesthetic such as lignocaine. A No. 1 needle is then inserted through this area into the dependent part of the cyst and the fluid content aspirated. The volume aspirated is measured and is replaced by a mixture of air and 25 per cent Hypaque. The volume of Hypaque used should not exceed 5 ml. The needle is removed and supero-inferior and medio-lateral views are taken. The aspirated fluid is retained; of this, part is examined histologically and part cultured.

Contraindications to the use of contrast examinations are sensitivity to the medium or infection within the breast, on the nipple or on the skin overlying the cystic lesion.

FLUIDOGRAPHY

Fluidography or isodensography (Dobretsberger, 1962; 1967) entails radiography with the breast suspended in 75–80 per cent alcohol. The alcohol and the breast have similar absorptive properties so that the contrast between the breast and surrounding air is eliminated with the result that all the structures from the nipple to the base of the breast may be seen clearly on one radiograph. A higher kilovoltage is used than with conventional mammography. Consequently the resultant mammogram has lower contrast than a conventional mammogram and fine microcalcification is not seen quite so clearly.

XERORADIOGRAPHY

This technique (Wolfe, 1968; 1969a) is similar to that of conventional mammography except for the fact that a xerographic plate is used instead of film. The plate is basically a sheet of aluminium coated with a layer of selenium enclosed in a cassette. The selenium is sensitized with an electrostatic charge. The breast is placed on the cassette and an x-ray exposure made. This leaves a residual charge pattern on the plate which is 'developed' by using oppositely charged coloured powder. The image is then transferred and fused onto a plastic coated paper.

One advantage of xeromammography is that the radiation dose to the patient is smaller because a higher kilovoltage and lower mAs values are used. Additionally the final xerographic image is similar to the conventional image but all edges are accentuated so that the normal structures and pathological lesions are more clearly demonstrated. Furthermore all structures from chest wall to nipple are well shown on the one plate and special viewing arrangments are not required. An excellent example of this technique is shown in *Figure 1.3* in which an occult carcinoma is demonstrated. The advantages of the technique are clearly illustrated.

70 MM PHOTOFLUOROGRAPHY

Basically this technique uses an Odelca system adapted for mammography (Gravelle, 1969). The unit has a Mullard Guardian 50 tube with 0·8 mm tungsten focus and incorporates a fine grain screen. The

13

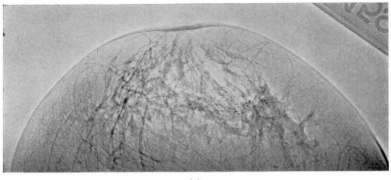

(a)

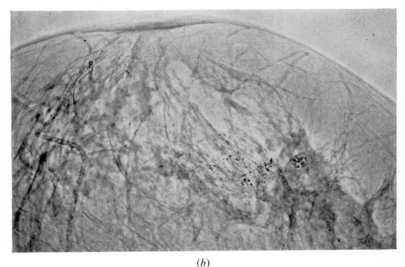

(b)

Figure 1.3. (a) Xeroradiograph showing an occult carcinoma. Supero-inferior view. Microcalcification is present in a spiculated lesion. The ducts are clearly shown; (b) detail of the irregular malignant lesion showing microcalcification and trabecular distortion. The calcification can be seen extending along ducts

(Reproduced by courtesy of Dr. J. N. Wolfe.)

screen image of the breast is recorded on 70 mm photographic film. Film may be exposed in lengths of 100 ft before processing or smaller lengths may be removed and processed separately. The factors used are 30–34 kV and 70 mAs. The unit is mounted on a motorized

14

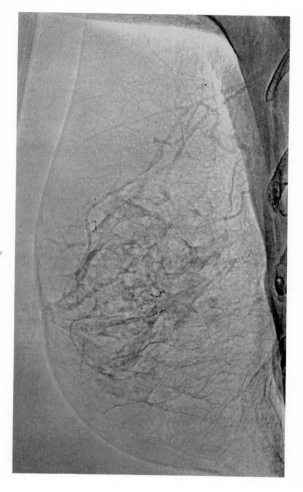

Figure 1.3 (cont.) (c) *Medio-lateral projection showing all structures from chest wall to nipple clearly. The veins and a calcified artery are well demonstrated*

(Reproduced by courtesy of Dr. J. N. Wolfe.)

stand and the camera and tube may be rotated so that supero-inferior and medio-lateral views can be obtained with the patient in the erect position.

The unit was designed with the possibility of mass surveys in mind. Large numbers can be examined quickly and relatively cheaply by means of this apparatus and its suitability in this respect has already been reported (Furnival *et al.*, 1970).

15

Chapter 2

Interpretation of Mammograms

I—The Normal Breast
Solitary and Multiple Smooth Lesions

An essential prerequisite to an accurate interpretation of mammograms is the production of radiographs of satisfactory quality. To attempt to give an opinion of inadequate films is to court disaster because an erroneous impression of security may be given. Films of the highest technical quality with respect to positioning and exposure are essential in order to show the detail that is so important in diagnosing or excluding breast cancer.

Full clinical information should be available in every case because this investigation is a complementary procedure to clinical examination. It is most important to know the exact position and clinical size of any palpable mass. It is helpful if all dominant masses are marked by means of lead markers. Naturally these marked areas should be examined closely but all areas of both breasts in all projections should be examined equally assiduously because a non-palpable malignant lesion may be present in a breast containing a benign palpable mass. Alternatively, in a patient who presents with a benign or a malignant lesion in one breast, an impalpable carcinoma may occur in the contralateral breast.

NORMAL FEMALE BREAST TYPES

It is essential to be familiar with the normal mammographic appearances which vary with the stage of development of the breast, with the patient's age and with the stage of the menstrual cycle.

The normal breast types fall mainly into four groups depending on the patient's age but there is considerable overlap in the appearances.

16

Normal Immature Breast

The immature or adolescent breast presents a more or less homo-geneous dense opacity in the glandular region (*Figure 2.1*). There is little infiltration of this region with fat and hence the dense appear-ance on the radiograph. The lactiferous ducts are not visible. Veins in the breast are faintly seen and occasionally trabeculae appear in late adolescence and the early part of the third decade. The compact dense glandular tissue contrasts well with the surrounding fatty tissue in the subcutaneous and retro-mammary regions which sepa-rate the gland from the skin and chest wall. The homogeneous glandular area is contiguous with the areola and nipple but where it borders on subcutaneous and retro-mammary fat the surface is

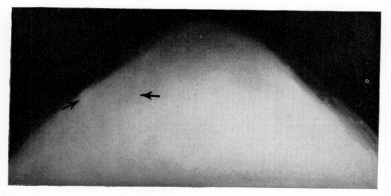

Figure 2.1. Immature adolescent breast. There is a homogeneous density of the whole gland. No trabeculae seen but veins faintly visible (arrowed).

(Reproduced from Evans and Gravelle (1969), by courtesy of the Editor, *X-ray Focus*.)

smooth and unbroken except where the delicate Cooper's suspensory ligaments occur. Homogeneous dense breasts are normal in adoles-cence and in the early twenties but such an appearance in the latter part of the third decade and early fourth decade is indicative of fibroadenosis. In this age group there is an increasing incidence of breast cancer and consequently malignancy may be obscured by the dense glandular tissue in such patients.

It is pertinent to state that not all adolescent breasts show homo-geneous glandular tissue. In some instances, even in early adolescence, a remarkable amount of fatty tissue is seen within the glandular area. The appearances are then indistinguishable from those of a mature glandular breast mammographically.

Normal Mature Breast

The mature adult breast, normally seen during the reproductive period, differs from the adolescent breast. Mammographically, there is both a reduction in the density of the glandular portion of the breast and an increased and variable amount of fat dispersed around

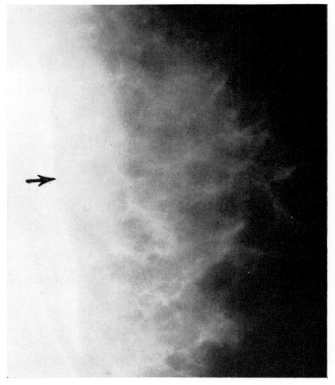

Figure 2.2. Mature adult breast. Fat is dispersed in the parenchyma and trabeculae are well seen. Note the retro-mammary fat line (arrowed)

the lobules of the breast parenchyma (*Figure 2.2*). Consequently appearances vary in the normal adult and mature breast depending on the relative amounts of fat and glandular tissue present. There is a variable irregular density with maximum density in the upper outer quadrant. The margins of the glandular portion are irregular with crescentic fatty incursions into the glandular mass. The veins are more easily seen than in the immature breast and trabeculation is now

18

prominent. In addition lactiferous ducts are more easily identified. Sub-areolar fat is almost invariably present and consequently the areola is clearly demonstrated. The amount of subcutaneous and retro-mammary fat is increased and as a result the skin is clearly shown around the whole breast. It should be noted that on the medio-lateral projection the skin over the inferior part of the breast may appear thickened. This is not true skin thickening but a radiographic

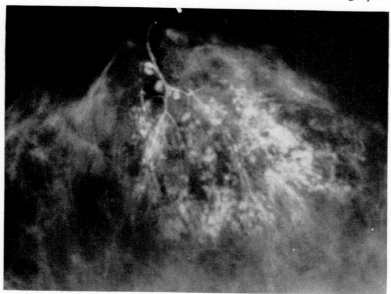

Figure 2.3. Lobular filling during contrast examination

illusion due to skin creasing. The true situation may be realized by comparison with the contralateral medio-lateral projection or by repeating the exposure following meticulous positioning. The areola is normally thicker than the adjoining skin and again comparison with the contralateral breast will help to decide whether or not there is pathological thickening in the areolar region.

The normal lactiferous ducts are not usually well demonstrated in conventional mammography of the mature breast. It is necessary to outline the ducts with a contrast medium to demonstrate the structures clearly.

There are 15–20 lactiferous ducts opening by separate ostia on the summit of the nipple. Immediately beneath the summit and within the substance of the nipple the ducts are narrow and take a straight course. The main ducts dilate beneath the areola to form the lactiferous sinuses. Beyond the sinuses the ducts again become narrow. The lobar ducts divide repeatedly into smaller and narrower ducts draining the lobules of the mammary gland. Occasionally the smallest lobules may be shown, particularly on over-filling during injection (*Figure 2.3*).

The Breast during Pregnancy

Following the onset of pregnancy the glandular portion of the breast becomes increasingly dense and this is associated with a loss of definition of the parenchyma and trabeculae. The intra-glandular fat becomes less obvious and the breast assumes an overall fluffiness with

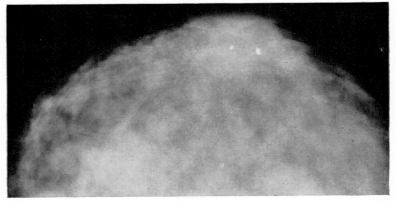

Figure 2.4. Late pregnancy. There is increased density, duct enlargment and marked lobular development

poor contrast. As the glandular portion of the breast enlarges it compresses the subcutaneous fat. The veins become larger and the lactiferous ducts also enlarge and become tortuous. Near term rounded opacities appear and are most noticeable in the sub-areolar region. They closely resemble cysts or fibroadenomas but actually represent saccules which are ordinarily too small to be seen but which become dilated and filled with milk in late pregnancy (*Figure 2.4*).

Following parturition the appearances remain largely unchanged except that the ducts become more prominent during lactation; the ducts and saccules vary in size, however, according to the volume of milk present. Involution following lactation is a slow and often irregular process. The ducts become progressively narrower and less tortuous but often a return to the pre-pregnant state is not obtained. Slight dilatation of the ducts following pregnancy may be accepted as

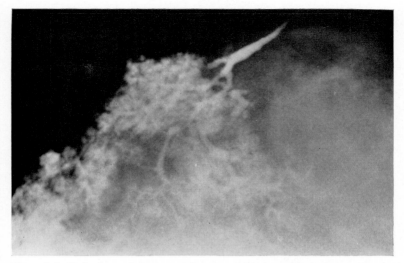

Figure 2.5. Slight duct enlargement and increased lobular development during pregnancy

a normal finding but the mammographic picture of the glandular portion on the whole returns to its original pattern.

The appearances of the ducts during pregnancy are shown in *Figure 2.5*. It is seen that the ducts are a little dilated and there is well marked lobular development. On the other hand duct injection shortly before term shows that the lactiferous ducts are markedly dilated and a saccule is also demonstrated (*Figure 2.6*).

The Post-menopausal Breast

As the menopause approaches the breast as a whole shrinks and the glandular portion involutes. In fatty breasts the relative proportion of fat to parenchyma increases and usually there is an actual increase in the amount of fat. This accentuates the natural contrast of the breast so that even small lesions can be clearly seen. As a result the trabeculae appear more prominent even though they become progressively thinner and the lactiferous ducts also stand out against the translucent fat. With advancing years the glandular portion is progressively replaced by fat giving a fatty atrophic breast with thin spidery trabeculae without glandular tissue but with faint opacification in the sub-areolar region due to the lactiferous ducts. Frequently there is arterial calcification also (*Figure 2.7*).

If little fat is present or if involution is incomplete there may be a relative increase in the amount of fibrous tissue so that the glandular

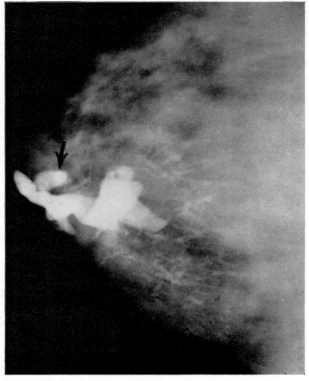

Figure 2.6. Marked duct dilatation in pregnancy shortly before delivery. A saccule is shown

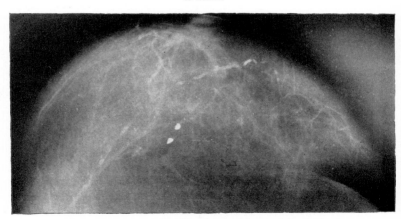

Figure 2.7. Fatty atrophic breast. There is arterial calcification
(Reproduced from Evans and Gravelle (1969), by courtesy of the Editor, *X-ray Focus*.)

portion of the breast appears as a dense area. Involution may produce a nodular appearance mainly in the upper outer quadrant and sub-areolar regions. This is a common finding although it is not strictly a normal appearance but is due to nodular fibrosis as a result of pre-existing fibroadenosis.

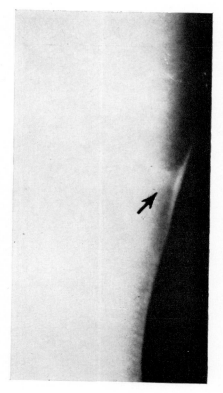

Figure 2.8. Normal male breast. Rudimentary glandular tissue is shown

THE NORMAL MALE BREAST

The normal male breast consists mainly of fat with the rudiments of glandular tissue seen faintly as a few small strands immediately beneath the nipple; a vein is usually clearly seen (*Figure 2.8*).

THE ABNORMAL BREAST

The radiographic appearances of the various pathological lesions encountered in breast disease will be superimposed on the normal features described in the preceding section. It is vital to distinguish malignant conditions from benign disease. There are several signs which will assist in this task but it is important to understand that the technique is not infallible. The radiographic signs of malignant and benign disease are set out in Table 2.1.

TABLE 2.1

Radiographic signs of malignancy	Radiographic signs of benignity
Direct signs	
1. Dense opacity (*a*) Irregular outline (*i*) Spicules (*ii*) Tentacles (*b*) Smooth outline—uncommon (*c*) Mixed outline—common (*d*) Diffuse breast opacification— fairly common 2. Microcalcification Fine and irregular Coarse and irregular	1. Low density opacity (*a*) Smooth outline (*i*) Circular or ovoid (*ii*) Lobulated (*b*) Ill-defined outline—occasional (*c*) Mixed outline—uncommon (*d*) Diffuse breast opacification— uncommon 2. Microcalcification Coarse and smooth Fine and smooth
Indirect signs	
1. Leborgne's Law Clinical size greater than radiographic size 2. Usually solitary lesion 3. Hypervascularity—common 4. Peri-focal haziness—common 5. Alteration of architecture— destruction of trabeculae 6. Alteration of breast outline— common	1. Leborgne's Law Clinical size equal to or less than radiographic size 2. Usually multiple lesions 3. Hypervascularity—fairly common 4. Peri-focal haziness—in inflammatory lesions 5. Alteration of architecture— displacement of trabeculae 6. Alteration of breast outline— fairly common

Several of the signs are common to both malignant and benign lesions. Consequently the correlation of signs and the pattern of breast involvement, together with knowledge of the clinical presentation and findings on examination, are crucial in leading to the correct diagnosis. It will be appreciated that if previous radiographs are available for comparison small changes may be more readily recognized.

The radiological signs may be classified as direct and indirect.

Radiological Signs: Direct

There are two direct signs—the presence of an opacity and microcalcification. These may be present alone or in combination. The density of a malignant lesion is usually much greater than that of the surrounding breast tissue. Benign lesions on the other hand are usually of low density and may even be transradiant.

Dense opacity.—The dense malignant opacity usually has an irregular outline which may show spicules or tentacles. A completely smooth outline is an uncommon finding in malignancy but lesions with outlines that are partly smooth and partly irregular are quite common. Diffuse breast involvement by carcinoma is also common. A benign lesion usually has smooth margins whether it is circular, ovoid or lobulated in outline but occasionally such a lesion may be ill-defined and uncommonly may show a mixed smooth and irregular outline. Diffuse breast opacification is uncommon in benign conditions.

Calcification.—Intra-mammary calcification if present is in most cases an accurate indication of the nature of the underlying pathology but this is not always the case, as will be discussed later. The more florid types of malignant and benign calcification are easily recognized and are invariably correct pointers to benign or malignant disease. The sparse, fine microcalcification usually gives rise to ambiguity but this is perhaps not surprising as in these cases there is often difficulty in deciding histologically whether the condition represents advanced epithelial hyperplasia or early intra-duct cacinoma. In general, malignant microcalcification is fine and irregular but occasionally it is coarse and irregular whereas benign calcification is often coarse and smooth and occasionally fine and smooth. Various reports (Leborgne and Dominguez, 1951; Egan, 1960; Gershon-Cohen *et al.*, 1962; Black and Young, 1965) place the incidence of characteristic microcalcification in malignant disease as seen on mammography at 30–40 per cent. Shepard *et al.* (1962) give an incidence of 75 per cent when paraffin blocks of breast carcinoma are examined radiographically but Black and Young (1965) are of the opinion that this higher incidence may be partly due to radiographic artefacts.

Radiological Signs: Indirect

Indirect radiographic signs are important as they indicate the possibility of malignancy and therefore lead to an even more thorough and detailed search of the mammograms. However it is important to realize that most of the indirect signs are present in benign as well as malignant disease.

Leborgne's Law.—A valuable indirect sign of malignancy is the result of an observation by Leborgne (1953) that the radiographic size of a malignant lesion is usually smaller than the clinical size of that lesion. The discrepancy in sizes may be explained on the grounds that a malignant lesion usually has an area of surrounding oedema which is clinically palpable but not always radiographically demonstrable. In using this sign care should be taken that the maximum

25

diameter of the tumour is measured on both the supero-inferior view and the medio-lateral projection. The measurement on the film and the clinical measurement should be carried out as shown in *Figure 2.9*. To obtain accurate results careful clinical and radiographic measurement is essential. In benign disease the clinical palpable mass is the same size or smaller than the lesion measured on the radiograph. The clinical size may be found to be smaller than the radiographic size of the lesion because a lax cyst is easily compressible clinically and so more difficult to measure accurately. Compression of the breast may alter the shape of the cyst so that it appears enlarged.

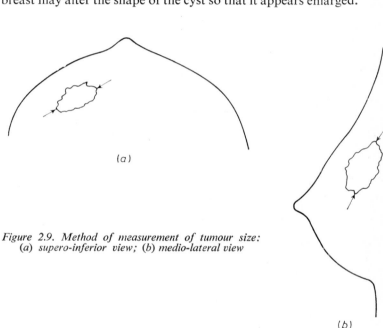

(a)

(b)

Figure 2.9. Method of measurement of tumour size: (a) supero-inferior view; (b) medio-lateral view

A malignant lesion is usually solitary and unilateral but may be multi-focal or bilateral. In addition a solitary malignant lesion or multi-focal lesions are often associated with benign lesions. In the majority of cases benign lesions are multiple and bilateral but can be solitary and unilateral.

Vascular changes.—Enlargement of the veins is a very common finding in a breast affected by malignant disease but it is not an invariable finding. Hypervascularity is usually found in acute and chronic breast abscesses and in infective and chemical mastitis. It may also occur in fibroadenosis and in association with fibroadeno- mas and with cysts. Infected cysts will always be associated with hypervascularity and recent haemorrhage into a cyst will usually be accompanied by venous engorgement. In addition asymmetry of the vein size is common in normal breasts, the left breast usually pos- sessing larger veins than the right. The presence of larger veins in the right breast should arouse great suspicion of malignancy.

Peri-focal haziness.—On close inspection it is often found that a malignant lesion has a surrounding zone of haziness which is not due to radiographic unsharpness but is the result of peri-focal oedema and collagenosis (Ingleby and Gershon-Cohen, 1960). Much of this oedema is invisible on the radiograph and it is the invisible portion that gives rise to the findings postulated in Leborgne's Law. How- ever, peri-focal haziness may be seen even though it may not be measurable. It is unusual to find a malignant lesion with borders well defined throughout its circumference. There is usually an area that is ill-defined. Rarely an encapsulated malignant tumour is seen which has completely smooth margins and even a surrounding zone of compressed fatty tissue giving a well demonstrated zone of trans- radiancy around the tumour. In such cases the lesion is usually a mucoid carcinoma or intra-cystic malignancy. The transradiant zone of com- pressed adipose tissue around a smooth lesion is known as a 'halo' and it is usually a good sign because in the vast majority of cases it indicates that the lesion is benign with no malignant infiltration of the surrounding fat. Even in the rare instances when a 'halo' sur- rounds a malignant lesion it is an indication that the tumour is encapsulated. Peri-focal haziness is not an infallible sign of malig- nancy because it may occur in breast abscess and other inflammatory breast diseases such as plasma cell mastitis.

Alterations in breast architecture and contour.—Both malignant and benign lesions may alter the architecture of the breast. Enlarge- ment of lactiferous ducts may occur in the neighbourhood of malig- nant lesions (Wolfe, 1967; 1969b) and may be the only feature in malignancy (*Figure 2.10*). The ducts may be straightened or tortuous. In benign disease duct ectasia may be the result of secretory disease or papillomatosis. A minor degree of duct ectasia may be regarded as an end result of pregnancy. Generalized or localized skin thickening is commonly found in malignancy and in benign inflammatory lesions. Areolar thickening may also occur in these conditions. Loss of clarity of the subcutaneous and retro-mammary fat may be due to malignant infiltration with oedema and collagenosis or to oedema as the result of inflammatory disease. Malignancy or inflammation can

27

produce either intra-mammary or axillary lymph gland enlargement, together with trabecular thickening and prominence of Cooper's ligaments. It is most important to note the effect a mass in the breast has on trabeculae; in malignancy there may be straightening or destruction of trabeculae in the neighbourhood of the lesion whereas with benign masses they are displaced rather than destroyed.

The contour of the breast will be affected by large malignant and benign masses and although nipple retraction is a well known sign of malignancy it occurs frequently in duct ectasia.

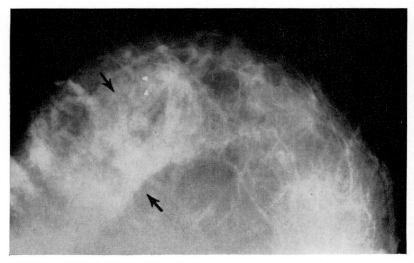

Figure 2.10. Enlarged ducts in non-infiltrative papilliferous intra-duct carcinoma

Examination of Radiographs

In examining mammograms it is useful to have a set routine so that all structures are examined on every occasion. The type of breast should be noted—whether it is immature, glandular, involutional or atrophic. A suitable point at which to commence the examination is the outer half of the breast in the supero-inferior projection. In all but atrophic breasts the amount of glandular tissue will be greatest in the outer half and in particular in the upper outer quadrant. A lesion is therefore more likely to be concealed here than elsewhere. Careful scanning using a variable light intensity is advisable. The inner half of the breast should next be examined. When examining the glandular portion the distribution of the trabeculae should be noted and the ducts identified if possible. The sub-areolar region and nipple are next examined noting particularly the thickness of the areola and skin. The subcutaneous fat is scrutinized for loss of transradiancy, for prominent Cooper's ligaments and also for extending spicules or tentacles. Axillary glands may be noted on the axillary tail view. As much as possible of the retro-mammary fat is examined at the same time. Finally the number and size of veins are noted. The contralateral supero-inferior view is examined in the same way and then both are viewed together so as to detect differences in density, skin thickening and hypervascularity. The same pattern of inspection is used for the medio-lateral projections and the axillae are further examined for lymph glands on these views.

When a lesion is present the important points to be noted are its density, shape, outline and position. The density should be compared with the density both of the glandular tissue and of any accompanying lesions. Inspection of the lesion and its surroundings for the presence of microcalcification is the next step and this is followed by a check on associated indirect signs. If there is any doubt as to the nature of the lesion then an accurate estimation of the clinical size should be obtained so that it can be compared with the radiographic size and Leborgne's law applied.

The abnormal radiographic features as they present in practice will be discussed. Abnormalities within the breast may be single or multiple. The lesions may be smooth or irregular and a diffuse abnormality may be present. The skin, nipple or ducts may be the site of pathological processes and intra-mammary calcification is an important feature in benign and malignant conditions.

THE SOLITARY SMOOTH LESION

Many conditions may present as a solitary smooth lesion and these can be classified according to the density of the opacity produced on the mammogram as summarized in Table 2.2.

Circumscribed Carcinoma

The most characteristic feature of a circumscribed carcinoma is its great density. It may be circular, ovoid or lobulated in shape and occasionally completely smooth with a surrounding halo but usually, on careful inspection, one ill-defined area will be found (*Figure 2.11*). The encapsulated type of tumour will displace trabeculae rather than destroy them but hypervascularity may be present. Peri-focal haziness and slight localized skin thickening should be sought, together with evidence of microcalcification. In the lobulated variety the indentations of the lobulation are broad and obtusely angled. There is a similar finding in a lobulated fibroadenoma. Circumscribed carcinomas may produce solitary smooth lesions of moderate density as well

TABLE 2.2
Solitary Smooth Lesion

Dense opacity	Moderately dense opacity
Circumscribed carcinoma	Circumscribed carcinoma
Intra-cystic papillary carcinoma	Cyst
Intra-cystic haemorrhage	Chronic abscess
Haematoma	Discrete adenosis
Giant fibroadenoma and Cystosarcoma	Fat necrosis
phylloides	Galactocoele
Large fibroadenoma	
Sarcoma	
Lymphosarcoma	
Infection—tuberculous cold abscess and	
Echinococcal cyst	
Metastatic deposit	

Low density opacity	Transradiant lesion
Fibroadenoma	Lipoma
Papilloma	Galactocoele
Cystic dilatation of a duct	Fat necrosis
Lymph gland	
Unilateral gynaecomastia	

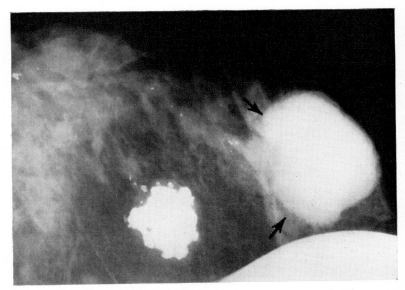

Figure 2.11. A dense smooth circumscribed carcinoma with an ill-defined area on its margin. A calcified fibroadenoma and benign microcalcification are present also
(Reproduced from Evans and Gravelle (1969), by courtesy of the Editor, *X-ray Focus*.)

as of great density. The features are identical with those previously described except that the density of the mass is not as great. These lesions are frequently mucoid carcinomas and present a mammographic and clinical problem because they may be quite soft on palpation. The presence of hypervascularity, localized haziness and skin thickening will help to indicate the true nature of the lesion but differentiation from a chronic abscess may be difficult.

Intra-cystic Papillary Carcinoma and Intra-cystic Haemorrhage

These may give appearances identical to those of circumscribed carcinoma. Mammographic recognition of intra-cystic haemorrhage may be possible on consideration of the clinical history and is more likely if previous films are available. Enlargement and increase in density of a pre-existing cyst would then be expected.

Haematoma

A history of trauma is usually available here but the trauma may be negligible in patients receiving anticoagulant therapy. The condition may be a complication of drill biopsy or open breast biopsy.

A haematoma is a dense, smooth, ovoid or rounded mass, displacing breast structures (*Fig. 2.12*). The overlying skin may be thickened

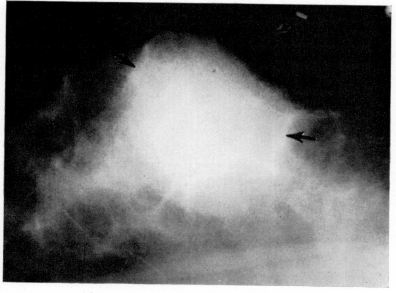

Figure 2.12. A haematoma displacing trabeculae

due to bruising or previous surgery. The lesion becomes gradually smaller eventually leaving either a small fibrotic area or no evidence of its previous existence. At the time of presentation the surrounding breast tissue may be a little hazy due to contusion and oedema.

Giant Fibroadenoma and Cystosarcoma Phylloides

There is some confusion in the nomenclature and interpretation of these conditions. Some authors use these terms synonymously and

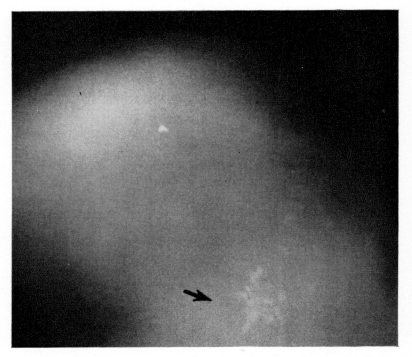

Figure 2.13. Coarse irregular flake-like calcification in cystosarcoma phylloides. Increased penetration is necessary to demonstrate this in the dense tumour

others use the term cystosarcoma to denote a malignant lesion whilst others again regard the condition as benign. Cystosarcoma is a cystic fleshy tumour which may be benign or malignant. It may be distinguished from giant fibroadenoma histologically but rarely on mammography. When coarse flake-like calcification is present it usually indicates that the lesion is cystosarcoma and not giant fibroadenoma (*Figure 2.13*). The term giant fibroadenoma should be used to denote a benign tumorous condition of the breast. Here again there is some difficulty in that the basis of differentiation from fibroadenoma is histological and not morphological. Giant fibroadenomas are not necessarily very large and may be smaller than fibroadenomas and, indeed, some fibroadenomas may in fact be much larger than giant fibroadenomas.

The giant fibroadenoma is usually a massive tumour which often occupies most of the breast, causing enlargement and alteration of breast outline. The breast parenchyma is displaced and compressed. The tumour is very dense and has a bosselated outline. The density is not completely homogeneous because faint linear and curvilinear semi-transradiancies may be seen and these represent the margins of the cotyledons of the tumour. Hypervascularity is invariably present but this may be exceedingly difficult to demonstrate owing to the dense nature of the tumour. In the uncomplicated case there is no skin thickening. On the contrary the skin is stretched and thin over the tumour and ulceration may occur. Superadded infection will then give oedema. Leborgne's law for benign tumours holds (*Figure 2.14*).

The smaller variety of giant fibroadenoma will have a similar appearance but the cotyledons will not be as large (*Figure 2.15*). The mass is dense and has many lobes with deep interstices so that the angles between the lobulations are more acute than in an ordinary fibroadenoma. Again hypervascularity is likely to be present and

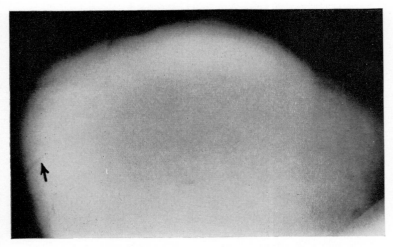

Figure 2.14. Giant fibroadenoma. The margins of the cotyledons may be seen faintly

33

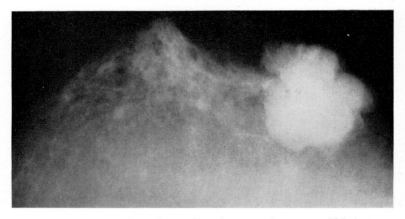

Figure 2.15. A relatively small giant fibroadenoma with pronounced lobulations

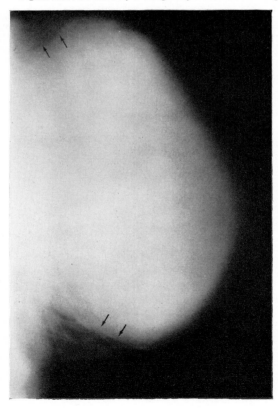

Figure 2.16. A large fibroadenoma occupying most of the breast and displacing breast structures

there will be displacement of breast structures but no peri-focal haziness or skin thickening. The radiographic size will be the same as the clinical size.

Large Fibroadenoma

An ordinary fibroadenoma is not usually radiopaque but if the tumour is very large then it becomes dense by virtue of its bulk. A large fibroadenoma will be very similar in appearance to a giant fibroadenoma but the divisions between the lobulations are not usually so deep as with the giant variety although a large fibroadenoma can be indistinguishable radiographically from a giant fibroadenoma (*Figure 2.16*). There will be hypervascularity, displacement of structures and alteration of breast outline. The clinical size will be the same as the radiographic size.

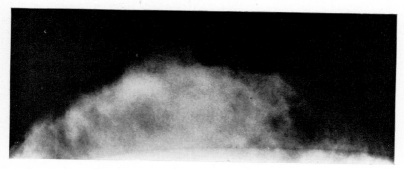

Figure 2.17. Angiosarcoma. There is a diffuse infiltrative lesion of the breast

Sarcoma

This is a rare neoplasm and the term should be confined to malignant varieties such as fibrosarcoma, adenosarcoma, carcinosarcoma, spindle cell sarcoma, chondrosarcoma, osteosarcoma and liposarcoma (Kennedy and Biggart, 1967). Angiosarcoma may be added to this list. Berger and Gershon-Cohen (1962) have described the appearances in breast sarcoma. The lesion is very dense with well-defined smooth margins and shows rapid growth with displacement of neighbouring structures rather than destruction. Cases of sarcoma originating in fibroadenomas may occur. They may resemble the appearances of giant fibroadenoma and cystosarcoma phylloides very closely. Some sarcomas produce dense diffuse lesions of the breast rather than localized tumours (*Figure 2.17*).

Lymphosarcoma

A lymphosarcoma is not strictly an example of breast sarcoma but can give rise to radiographic appearances that are identical with those of sarcomatous tumours of the breast.

Infection

Tuberculous cold abscess and echinococcal cyst are both rare infections of the breast that give rise to solitary dense smooth lesions. Examples of both conditions have been illustrated by Leborgne (1953). They present no characteristic features.

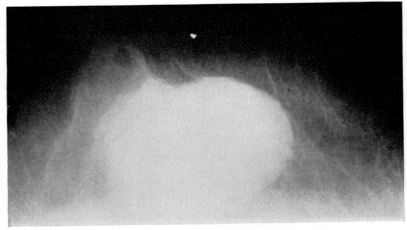

Figure 2.18. A solitary cyst slightly lobulated and displacing trabeculae

Metastatic Deposit

A metastatic deposit from a primary tumour elsewhere in the body —e.g., bronchogenic carcinoma or melanoma—may give a smooth, rounded, dense opacity which may be mistaken for a circumscribed carcinoma.

Cyst

Cysts are the commonest lesions of the breast but they are usually multiple and present in both breasts. They may be rounded, ovoid or lobulated (*Figure 2.18*). Lobulation occurs in a multilocular cyst and an apparent lobulation may be due to the close proximity and the overlapping of several cysts (*Figure 2.19*). Cysts are variable in size and may vary in size quite markedly at different examinations. They are of homogeneous density and are relatively denser than the surrounding breast tissue. Infrequently marginal 'egg shell' calcification may occur but this is not pathognomonic *Figure 2.20*). Trabeculae in the neighbourhood of the lesion are displaced and the radiographic size may be the same or greater than the clinical size. The latter state of affairs occurs with lax cysts which may cause false small clinical measurements to be taken because the end points are difficult to determine and the cyst is easily compressible. In addition the laxity of the cyst may allow considerable distortion of the lesion in the various mammographic projections giving a false

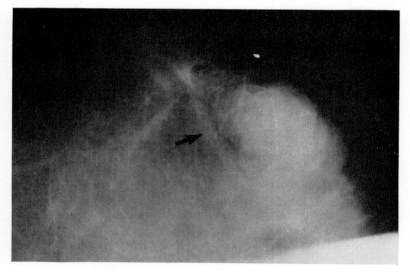

Figure 2.19. Overlapping cysts giving an impression of lobulation. There is displacement of ducts and trabeculae

large radiographic measurement. Normally there will be no hypervascularity but if the cyst is inflamed then there may be venous engorgement and even peri-focal haziness and skin thickening. Cyst aspiration and replacement of the fluid with gas and an opaque medium is a certain method of diagnosing the presence of a cyst and in addition the benign nature of the cystic mass will be demonstrated with this technique (*Figure 2.21*). All cysts of whatever origin will have similar radiographic appearances. There will be variation in the density of the lesion according to the volume of fluid the lesion contains and also according to the nature of the fluid within the cyst. Haemorrhage into the cyst will cause an increase in density.

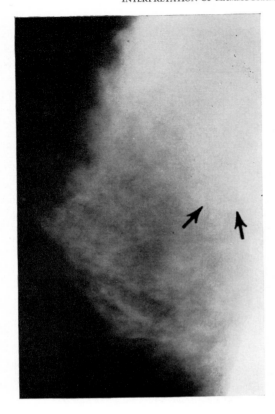

Figure 2.20. 'Egg-shell' calcification in the margin of a cyst

(Reproduced from Evans and Gravelle (1969), by courtesy of the Editor, *X-ray Focus*.)

Chronic Abscess

The longer the duration of a breast abscess the more localized it becomes so that a chronic abscess presents smooth margins. The lesion is circular or ovoid and usually of moderate density (*Figure 2.22*). It resembles a cyst and if localized oedema and hypervascularity are present it is difficult to distinguish from a circumscribed carcinoma as localized skin thickening is often present, except in small deeply situated abscesses. An occasional broad 'tentacle' is seen extending outwards into the parenchyma. The clinical history and findings are often helpful in indicating the true nature of the lesion. When the patient has received antibiotic therapy the perifocal oedema, skin thickening and hypervascularity may be negligible or even absent and then differentiation of such an 'antibioma' from a cyst is extremely difficult and usually impossible. If there is

38

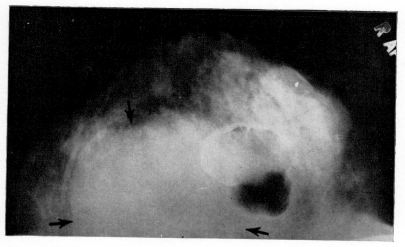

Figure 2.21. Contrast examination of a multi-locular cyst showing smooth inner walls. The adjacent large cyst was impalpable
(Reproduced from Evans and Gravelle (1969), by courtesy of the Editor, *X-ray Focus*.)

associated oedema the clinical size may be larger than the radiographic size.

Discrete Adenosis

Adenosis or lobular hyperplasia can be a physiological process but when it becomes excessive and symptomatic it may be regarded as pathological. Foci of adenosis are usually multiple and bilateral but changes may be predominantly in one breast and discrete giving rise to a smooth, rounded or ovoid opacity usually within an area of breast parenchyma showing homogeneous increase in density (*Figure 2.23*). The area of discrete adenosis is usually only slightly more dense than the surrounding breast tissue and it may be impossible both mammographically and clinically to distinguish it from a cyst or fibroadenoma. There may be hypervascularity but there will be no oedema or skin thickening and its clinical size will be the same as the radiographic size.

Fat Necrosis

Fat necrosis may be the result of trauma to the breast or secondary to plasma cell mastitis produced as a result of rupture of ectatic lactiferous ducts in secretory disease. The sequence is the same in both instances. A chemical mastitis occurs which results in necrosis of the neighbouring adipose tissue. The initial lesions are ill-defined

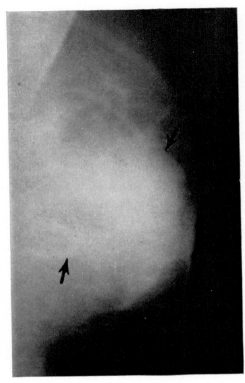

Figure 2.22. A chronic sub-areolar abscess. There is hypervascularity and areolar thickening. A broad tentacle is seen posteriorly

but as the inflammation resolves the area of fat necrosis becomes more localized and circumscribed eventually leaving a rounded, ovoid or lobulated smooth lesion (*Figure 2.24*). The lesion may become progressively smaller eventually leaving an area of fibrosis or it may become transradiant or calcified.

Galactocoele

A galactocoele arises in a lactating breast and may initially appear as a smooth, rounded moderately dense lesion situated in a breast showing the changes of pregnancy and lactation. It will therefore be impossible to distinguish between it and a cyst, fibroadenoma or dilated sub-areolar saccule at this stage. It may persist as an opaque lesion long after lactation has ceased but may also become trans-radiant (*Figure 2.25a, b*).

LOW-DENSITY, SOLITARY, SHARPLY-DEFINED LESIONS

A lesion is regarded as producing a low density opacity when the

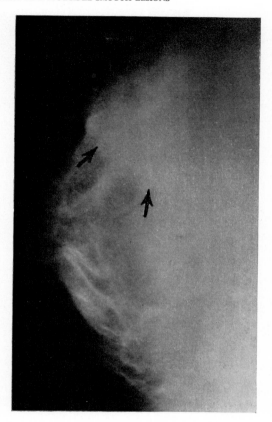

Figure 2.23. The smooth low density circumscribed lesion was an area of discrete adenosis

density of the lesion approximates that of the surrounding glandular tissue. The following conditions give a low density opacity.

Fibroadenoma

This is a very common tumour in the young at any age between 14 and 20 years and is occasionally seen in older women. It is usually solitary. Except when the tumour is large, its density is so similar to that of the surrounding breast tissue that it may be very difficult to detect. The only clue may be the presence of a smooth border silhouetted against the mammary fat (*Figure 2.26*). If the tumour is surrounded by a transradiant halo of compressed fat then its existence is clearly demonstrated (*Figure 2.27*). The tumour outline may be rounded or lobulated and occasionally ovoid. If it is lobulated, the

41

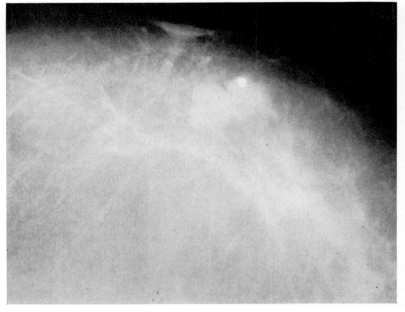

Figure 2.24. A lobulated lesion clinically thought to be malignant. Mammographically it was reported as benign. Histology showed fat necrosis

indentations are shallow and usually obtusely angled. The radiographic and clinical sizes are the same. Calcification may be present and this will accentuate the opacity of the lesion.

Papilloma

A solitary papilloma may give rise to a smooth, rounded or ovoid low density lesion (*Figure 2.28a*). It will not usually be differentiated from a cyst or fibroadenoma on mammography unless there is a history of blood-stained nipple discharge in the absence of a palpable lesion. Injection of the duct with contrast medium is usually required to confirm the plain film findings (*Figure 2.28b*). The presence of fine punctate calcification within the opacity may give an indication of the nature of the lesion.

Cystic Dilatation of a Duct

The mammographic appearances will be similar to those of papilloma and contrast studies will be required to elucidate them.

Lymph Gland

An intra-mammary lymph gland is frequently seen in the sub-

SOLITARY AND MULTIPLE SMOOTH LESIONS

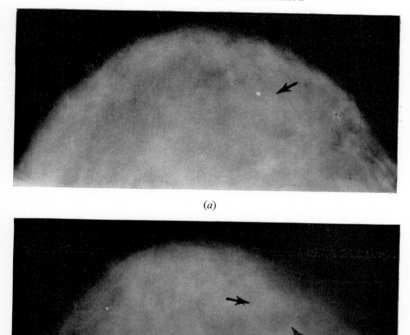

(a)

(b)

Figure 2.25. Galactocoele. (a) Breast during pregnancy with a smooth mobile lump. Low density lesion on mammography; (b) same case following delivery and artificial suppression of lactation. A transradiant lesion is now seen at the site of the lump

cutaneous fat in the region of the axillary tail and may also occur within the mammary glandular substance as well as in the axillary fat (*Figure 2.29*). The lymph gland is often ovoid with a notch in one margin and may resemble a fibroadenoma or cyst. The presence of a lymph gland may be a completely normal finding and does not necessarily indicate breast disease.

Unilateral Gynaecomastia

Gynaecomastia is frequently unilateral in distribution and as such may present radiographically as a solitary smooth lesion (*Figure 2.30*). Glandular structures may be faintly seen but if there is associated

43

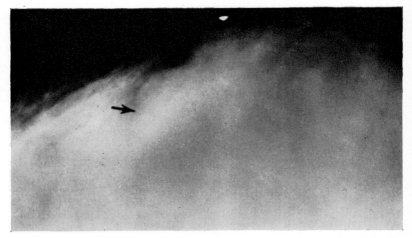

Figure 2.26. Fibroadenoma silhouetted against the subcutaneous fat. Its density is similar to that of the glandular tissue

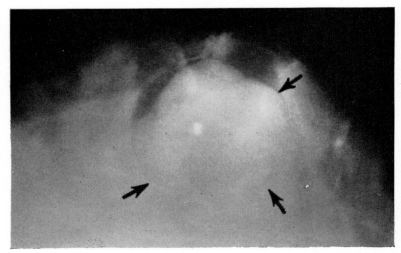

Figure 2.27. Lobulated fibroadenoma outlined by the transradiant fat 'halo'

mastitis then the opacity is homogeneous, smooth and rather tri-angular in shape.

TRANSRADIANT, SOLITARY, SHARPLY-DEFINED LESIONS

Lipoma

A lipoma is usually ovoid or lobulated, the margins of the lesion

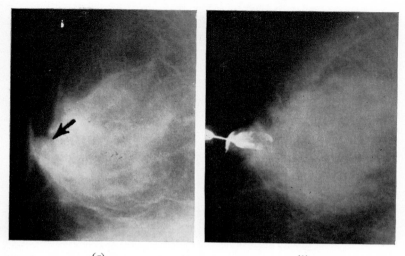

(a)   (b)

Figure 2.28. Papilloma. (a) A low density opacity is seen immediately beneath the nipple; (b) injection demonstrates the smooth lobulated papilloma

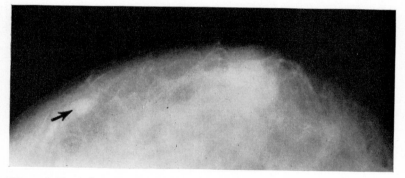

Figure 2.29. A few cysts are present and a normal lymph gland is also shown (histological proof). A small notch is present in it

being composed of displaced trabeculae (*Figure 2.31*). If the tumour occurs in a glandular breast then it stands out clearly on the radiograph. However, if it occurs in a fatty breast it will not be as clearly seen but the displacement of the trabeculae will draw the radiologist's attention to the fact that within the area encompassed by the displaced trabeculae there is increased transradiancy compared with that of the surrounding fat.

45

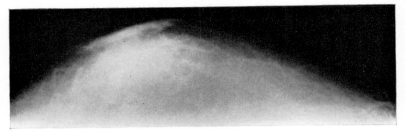

Figure 2.30. Unilateral gynaecomastia. A small triangular mass of glandular tissue is present immediately behind the nipple

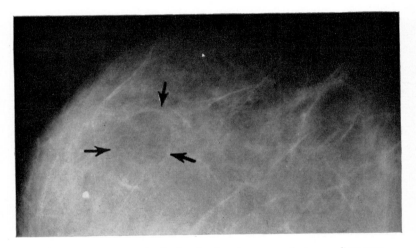

Figure 2.31. A lipoma. The displaced trabeculae surround a transradiant area

Galactocoele

The milk content of a galactocoele may undergo chemical change so that an opaque lesion changes to a non-opaque lesion presumably as the result of a high fat content. It may be possible to follow this transition radiographically or the galactocoele may be seen as a transradiant smooth, rounded lesion during the initial examination (*Figure 2.25a, b*).

Fat Necrosis

This condition may also give rise to a smooth, rounded transradiant lesion similar to a galactocoele. A change from an opaque to a non-opaque lesion may occur over a period of time. Leborgne (1953) has also illustrated a case of traumatic fat necrosis that originally showed a smooth transradiancy which after eighteen months became opaque but was otherwise unchanged. The margins of the lesion may ultimately become calcified.

MULTIPLE SMOOTH LESIONS

The breast diseases that give rise to multiple smooth lesions in the mammogram are shown in Table 2.3. Not only are the lesions multiple in one breast but they are often bilateral. They are mainly the same

TABLE 2.3
Multiple Smooth Lesions

Moderately dense opacities	Low density opacities
Cysts Fibroadenosis with cysts and fibroadenomas Fibroadenomas Lobular carcinoma Galactocoeles Fat necrosis	Fibroadenomas Papillomatosis Cystic duct ectasia
Transradiant lesions	Mixed transradiant and low density lesions
Lipomas Galactocoeles Fat necrosis	Fibroadenolipoma

lesions that give rise to the single smooth opacities described earlier, their radiographic appearances being unaltered by their multiplicity.

Cysts

As will be seen from the several examples demonstrated, cysts may vary enormously in number and size (*Figures 2.21* and *2.32*). Associated changes indicating the aetiological nature of the cyst may be present—i.e., the changes of duct ectasia will be present with secretory cysts and sebaceous and apocrine cysts will be closely related to the skin. Frequently, while only one cyst is clinically palpable, radiographically it is clear that there are very many present (*Figures 2.21* and *2.33*). The explanation is that the clinician feels only the tense superficial lesion while the soft lax cysts, whether they are superficial

47

or deep in position, have a similar texture to breast tissue and are therefore impalpable. In addition, it is usually the tension in the cyst that causes symptoms and so draws attention to its presence. Contrast examination is the only radiographic method that will demonstrate the interior of a cyst although increase in density of a cyst should arouse suspicion that there is either an intra-cystic papilloma or carcinoma, or that intra-cystic haemorrhage has occurred.

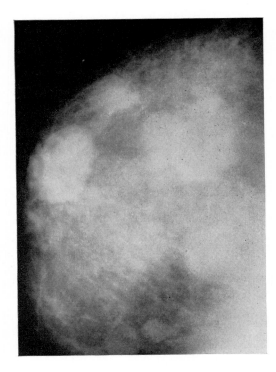

Figure 2.32. Multiple cysts of varying sizes

Generally, cysts are either ovoid or rounded but quite frequently they are lobulated (*Figures 2.18, 2.21* and *2.33*). Lobulation may be due to the fact that the cyst is multi-locular or that a number of cysts are arranged close to one another so that they overlap in the different projections. With a multi-locular cyst the angles of lobulation may be wide, as is the case with fibroadenomas. When lobulation is due to a collection of cysts the angles tend to be more acute.

Transradiant haloes are frequently seen around cysts and may completely or partially surround a single cyst or many cysts.

Leborgne's law holds in general, the clinical size being either the same as, or smaller than, the radiographic size. However, when the clinician palpates and measures a group of contiguous cysts the clinical measurement will be greater than the radiographic measurement of the individual cysts.

Fibroadenosis with Cysts and Fibroadenomas

Other terms used to denote this association are fibrocystic disease, chronic cystic mastitis and fibroadenomatosis. Most cystic disease of the breast is associated with fibroadenosis and this may be very evident on the radiographs or there may be little radiographic evidence of fibroadenosis. In the latter cases the cystic changes predominate and the cysts tend to be larger than in those cases in which

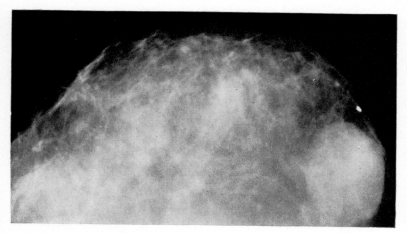

Figure 2.33. One dominant palpable cyst with numerous small impalpable cysts

fibroadenotic changes are obvious. A third group is also seen in which the fibroadenosis predominates and the cysts are only faintly visualized through the opacity due to the dense fibrosis.

Fibroadenosis produces a 'ground glass' increase in density in the glandular area of the breast and the margins of the area then assume a smoother appearance than is normal. Superimposed on this appearance and closely intermingled with the breast parenchyma numerous smooth, rounded opacities will be seen. These are usually small but variable in size. They are mainly cysts but fibroadenomas may be present together with hyperplastic fibrotic nodules. These

49

lesions will usually be indistinguishable on the radiograph (*Figure 2.34*). Occasionally a fibroadenoma will contain characteristic calcification and will then be easily recognizable (*Figure 2.35*).

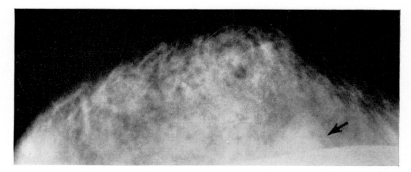

Figure 2.34. Fibroadenosis with cysts and fibroadenomas. There is a ground glass increase in density with numerous smooth, rounded lesions of varying size. The arrowed lesion was a fibroadenoma. The calcification of secretory disease is also present

A similar radiographic appearance may be found when fibroadenosis with cysts and fibroadenomas co-exists with secretory disease giving a condition known as Schimmelbusch's disease or mastopathy (*Figures 2.34* and *2.36*). It is said to occur when several dysplasias are present in the same breast. It differs radiographically from fibroadenosis with cysts and fibroadenomas because evidence of duct ectasia can be seen and frequently the characteristic calcification of burnt-out secretory disease is also present (*Figure 2.34*).

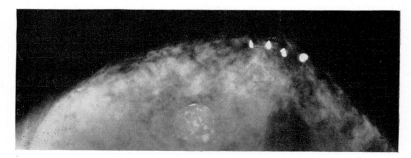

Figure 2.35. Fibroadenosis with cysts and a calcified fibroadenoma

Fibroadenomas

Usually moderately large multiple fibroadenomas will be indistinguishable from multiple cysts because their density may be greater than the surrounding breast tissue (*Figure 2.37*). The several separate tumours are more likely to be clinically palpable than cysts.

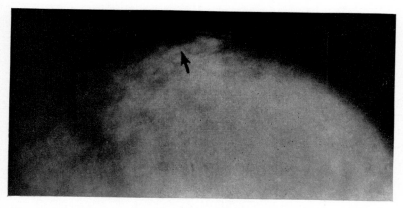

Figure 2.36. Schimmelbusch's mastopathy. Dilated ducts are present beneath the nipple and numerous cysts can be seen throughout the breast superimposed on the ground glass density of fibroadenosis

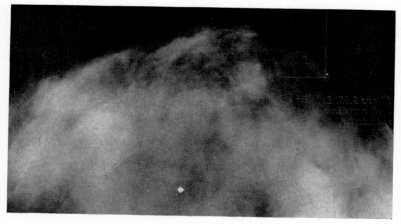

Figure 2.37. Multiple fibroadenomas indistinguishable from cysts

51

Lobular Carcinoma

This is an unusual type of malignant involvement in which there are multiple malignant foci either arising in, or spreading via, the lobules (Foote and Stewart, 1941). There may be little to indicate that the lesions are malignant except the presence of hypervascularity, skin thickening and oedema. The lesions may be smooth and of

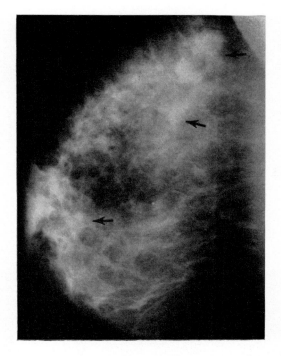

Figure 2.38. Lobular carcinoma. The appearances are very similar to fibroadenosis with cysts in this case. There are smooth rounded lesions but there is also hypervascularity, areolar thickening and diffuse increase in density with trabecular thickening

moderate density with no microcalcification (*Figure 2.38*); occasionally they may have ill-defined margins.

Galactocoeles and Fat Necrosis

Multiple opaque galactocoeles and multiple areas of fat necrosis will not differ from the solitary varieties in their radiographic appearances (*see* page 46).

Multiple smooth low density opacities would be expected with small fibroadenomas, papillomatosis and cystic duct ectasia. Small fibroadenomas will give rise to opacities similar to the solitary tumour. They are seldom numerous and may be calcified. Papillomatosis may be diagnosed radiographically in the presence of a beaded appearance of the lactiferous ducts in association with a

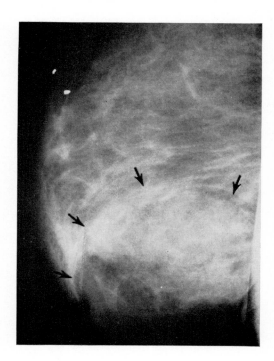

Figure 2.39. Fibroadeno-lipoma. The lesion consists of a mixture of lipomatous and fibroadenomatous tissues

history of nipple discharge, especially if the discharge is blood-stained. Fine punctate microcalcification may be present.

Cystic duct ectasia is rarely distinguishable from small cysts but may be considered if there is a history of serous, greenish or brown nipple discharge.

Multiple smooth transradiant lesions are uncommon but could be due to lipomas, fat necrosis or galactocoeles.

Fibroadenolipoma

This is an unusual lesion giving rise to multiple smooth opacities in conjunction with a transradiant zone which is lipomatous, the other opacities being due either to fibroadenosis or fibroadenomas or a combination of both (*Figure 2.39*) (Leborgne, 1953; Egan, 1970).

II—Solitary and Multiple Irregular Lesions

THE SOLITARY IRREGULAR LESION

The commonest cause of a solitary irregular breast lesion is a carcinoma. Other conditions giving rise to irregular opacities are tabulated in Table 2.4.

TABLE 2.4
Solitary Irregular Lesion

Dense opacity	Moderately dense opacity	Low density opacity
Carcinoma	Carcinoma Chronic abscess Plasma cell mastitis Sclerosing adenosis	Adenosis Fibroadenoma Acute abscess

Carcinoma

One of the most characteristic features of a malignant lesion is that it gives a dense opacity and the margins of the opacity are usually irregular. This combination of features enables a radiographic diagnosis of malignancy to be made in the majority of cases.

Several patterns of irregularity of outline occur. Radiating spicules, indicating the presence of a scirrhous reaction, are the commonest finding. The spicules may be either prominent and several centimetres long (*Figure 2.40*) or short and delicate (*Figure 2.41*). Some carcinomas possess thicker radiating tentacles of varying length (*Figures 2.42* and *2.43*). This form again occurs in the presence of a scirrhous reaction. Spicules and tentacles may co-exist.

The tumour outline may not necessarily be completely irregular; tumours with partly smooth and partly irregular margins are fairly common. These may show a smooth outline with tentacles arising at

55

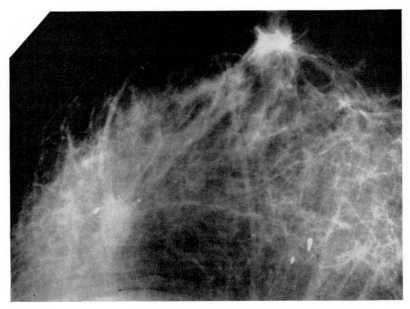

Figure 2.40. A dense scirrhous carcinoma with long spicules causing trabecular destruction. The calcification of secretory disease is present also and dilated ducts can be seen

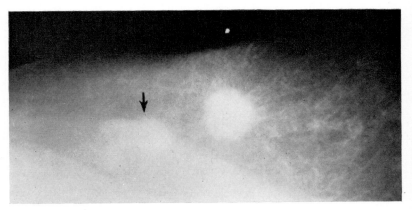

Figure 2.41. Scirrhous carcinoma with short fine spicules and enlarged axillary lymph nodes shown on the axillary tail projection

56

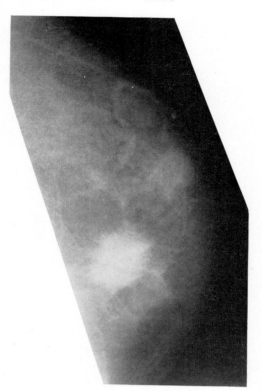

Figure 2.42. Scirrhous carcinoma with short thick tentacles and microcalcification which is partly within the tumour and partly outside the mass

(Reproduced from Evans and Gravelle (1969), by courtesy of the Editor, *X-ray Focus*.)

intervals. Alternatively the main bulk of the tumour may be smooth and a leash of spicules or tentacles arises to one side, usually following the line of the lactiferous ducts towards the nipple although they may be directed posteriorly. This gives rise to the so-called 'comet tail' appearance (*Figure 2.44*). A similar appearance may be found in association with a spiculated tumour (*Figure 2.45*).

Confirmatory microcalcification should always be sought and the secondary features of malignancy—especially thickening and destruction of trabeculae and peri-focal haziness—checked. The radiographic measurement should be less than the clinical measurement.

Breast carcinoma may occasionally give a moderately dense irregular radiographic opacity. If tentacles are present then differentiation from a chronic abscess may be extremely difficult on radiographic grounds alone.

Chronic Abscess

Although this lesion may exhibit a moderately dense opacity with an irregular outline in the form of extending processes and so may

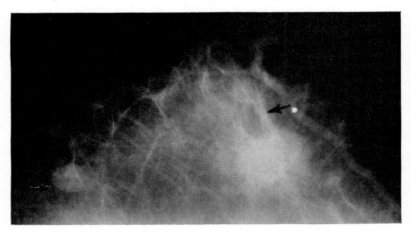

Figure 2.43. Scirrhous carcinoma with long thick tentacles destroying trabeculae. There is hypervascularity and an enlarged intra-mammary lymph node is present

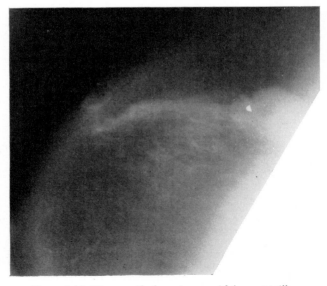

Figure 2.44. Circumscribed carcinoma with 'comet-tail'

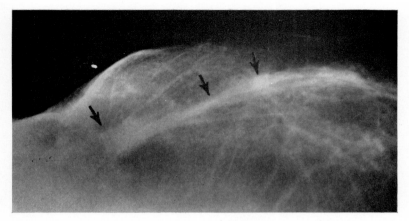

Figure 2.45. Spiculated carcinoma with 'comet-tail' extension to the nipple and overlying localized skin thickening

resemble a carcinoma closely, a distinction does occur. The processes are usually less numerous than the tentacles in malignancy and there is an absence of spiculation (*see Figure 2.22*). In addition, fine microcalcification does not occur in abscesses although an old healed abscess may show coarse calcification. If there is considerable oedema, Leborgne's law for benign lesions may not apply.

Plasma Cell Mastitis

Plasma cell mastitis is a complication of duct ectasia and secretory disease. With rupture of the duct and liberation of its secretions into the breast substance a foreign body inflammatory reaction is set up in response to the irritant properties of the duct contents. The inflammation usually results in pain and swelling with formation of a palpable mass.

The condition gives rise to a moderately dense irregular opacity (*Figures 2.46* and *2.48*). This may assume a variety of shapes but often in the later stages flame-like opacities extend from the involved ducts (*Figure 2.47*). In the acute phase the opacities are associated with localized oedema, skin or areolar thickening and venous engorgement. At this stage, the radiographic size may be smaller than the clinical size as a result of the localized oedema. There may be some difficulty therefore in distinguishing between active plasma cell mastitis and malignancy. Several features will assist in the differentiation. Plasma cell mastitis will occur in breasts with bilateral evidence of duct ectasia. Carcinoma of course often occurs in breasts affected by duct ectasia also (*see Figure 2.40*) but if there is no evidence of duct ectasia then this is a point in support of a diagnosis of carcinoma.

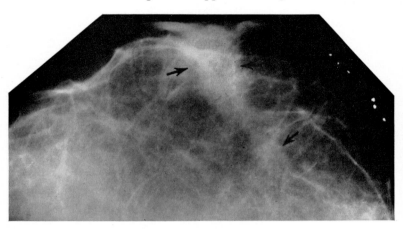

Figure 2.46. An area of plasma cell mastitis in the sub-areolar region diagnosed radiologically. The nipple is retracted and there is areolar oedema. Clinically this was considered to be a carcinoma. Dilated ducts are seen deep in the breast

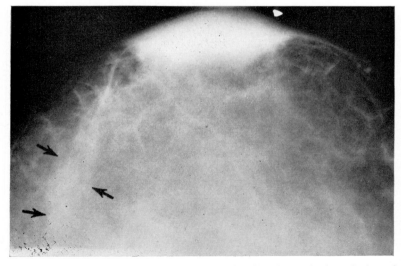

Figure 2.47. Plasma cell mastitis. There is a flame-shaped opacity along the line of the ducts and there is marked areolar oedema. Dilated ducts are faintly visible in the sub-areolar region

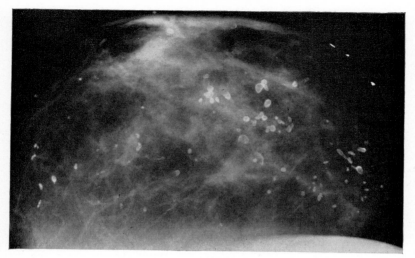

Figure 2.48. Plasma cell mastitis in the sub-areolar region with marked areolar oedema and adjacent skin thickening. There is widespread calcification of the type seen in burnt-out secretory disease

Trabecular thickening occurs in both conditions but the irregular marginal processes in plasma cell mastitis extend along the trabeculae while the spicules and tentacles of carcinoma frequently run across the line of the trabeculae and destroy them. The malignant opacity is usually denser than that of plasma cell mastitis and may contain characteristic calcification differing completely from the duct calcification of secretory disease.

Plasma cell mastitis frequently occurs in the sub-areolar region but may also occur elsewhere in the breast. Carcinoma may also be sub-areolar in position but it more commonly occurs within the breast parenchyma. Nipple retraction may be present in both conditions but is frequently bilateral in plasma cell mastitis as the underlying duct ectasia is bilateral and a common cause of nipple retraction. If the clinical size is the same as the radiographic size in acute plasma cell mastitis this is a good indication that a benign condition is present but if there is much surrounding oedema the radiographic size may be smaller than the clinical size. However, plasma cell mastitis frequently subsides in a few days with consequent reduction in the clinical size to that measured from the radiograph.

Following subsidence of the inflammation the opacity may disappear or a residual irregular fibrous area may remain which will

61

have none of the secondary signs of malignancy and no fine micro-calcification. It will conform to Leborgne's law.

Sclerosing Adenosis

Adenosis is a common mammographic finding and although it may be discrete it is more commonly widespread and bilateral even though the breasts may be affected unequally. The condition may wax and wane or resolve. It may also set up a reactive fibrous response in the breast leading to the formation of a localized hard mass which may be fixed. The association of adenosis with reactive fibrosis is known as sclerosing adenosis.

Sclerosing adenosis usually occurs on a background of adenosis but is included in this group of solitary irregular lesions because it is the dominant lesion in the radiograph (*Figure 2.49*). Its density is greater than that of the breast tissue and of the accompanying adenosis. The opacity may be stellate in shape and resemble a small carcinoma but there is no localized skin thickening even though clinically there may be a suggestion of this. It is usually peripherally situated and not sub-areolar in position. Venous engorgement is not a feature of sclerosing adenosis but may be present due to the accompanying adenosis. Distortion of trabeculae may occur as a result of the fibrosis

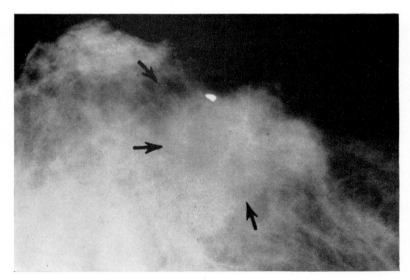

Figure 2.49. Sclerosing adenosis showing as an irregular dense area in a fibroadenotic breast

but there is no microcalcification and, most important of all, the clinical size is the same as the radiographic size.

Three conditions, adenosis, fibroadenoma and acute breast abscess may give solitary irregular radiographic lesions of low density.

Adenosis

Adenosis, although usually giving rise to multiple bilateral changes, may sometimes cause a solitary irregular low density lesion. The affected area will have a fluffy ground glass appearance. It may produce a palpable mass but radiographically there is usually no difficulty in distinguishing it from malignancy because it is of low density and without oedema or skin thickening. There may be hypervascularity but there is no trabecular disruption even though there may be trabecular thickening. However, the radiographic size of the lesion is the same as the clinical measurement.

Fibroadenoma

Part of the periphery of a fibroadenoma is frequently obscured or ill-defined because it lacks surrounding fat and is of the same density as the breast tissue (*see Figure 2.26*). In addition a recently developed fibroadenoma may not be completely encapsulated so that it will not possess a smooth margin where it emerges from an area of fibroadenosis. A third cause for loss of definition is the swelling and oedema of the tumour that may occur during the menstrual phase.

Acute Abscess

An acute abscess will give rise to a low density ill-defined opacity associated with trabecular thickening, peri-focal oedema, skin thickening and marked venous engorgement. It will not usually be possible to measure the areas involved in the radiograph due to the uncertainty of position of the margins of the abscess. In fact, the only change may be one of a slight increase in density as compared with the corresponding area of the contralateral breast.

The abscess may progress to generalized cellulitis or may become chronic when it becomes increasingly localized and more obvious radiographically.

MULTIPLE IRREGULAR LESIONS

These lesions are classified in Table 2.5.

TABLE 2.5

(a) Multiple Irregular Lesions

Dense opacities	Moderately dense opacities
Multifocal carcinoma	Multifocal carcinoma Plasma cell mastitis Sclerosing adenosis

(b) Co-existing Smooth and Irregular Lesions

1. Carcinoma with dysplasia
2. Schimmelbusch's mastopathy
3. Fibroadenosis with cysts

Multifocal Carcinoma

When dense multiple irregular lesions are found the diagnosis is practically always that of multifocal carcinoma. The lesions may be confined to one breast (*Figure 2.50*) or may be present in both breasts (*Figure 2.51a, b*). Multifocal malignant lesions may be bilateral and simultaneous or may occur in the contralateral breast following mastectomy, at varying periods from months to many years. Tumours developing in the contralateral breast over 5 years

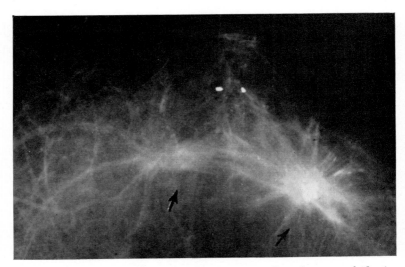

Figure 2.50. Two spiculated malignant foci are present. Smooth coarse calcification is present near one focus. This is due either to fat necrosis or a co-existing fibroadenoma

64

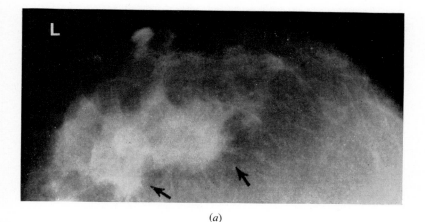

(a)

(b)

Figure 2.51. (a) and (b). Simultaneous bilateral breast carcinomas

after mastectomy are usually regarded as new primary lesions. This however is not necessarily the case, because metastases may occur after 5 years and secondary primary tumours may occur in less than 5 years.

It is not possible to differentiate primary tumours from metastatic deposits mammographically because both may have identical features. Egan (1970) has attempted to differentiate these lesions on mammographic appearances but none of the described features is typical of one type of tumour. He maintains that diffuse breast involvement without evidence of a mass is indicative of metastatic

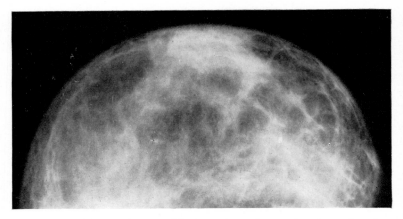

Figure 2.52. Diffuse involvement of the breast in carcinoma: the primary focus here is obscured by the increased density

disease. These features may occur in metastatic disease but identical appearances may also be seen in advanced primary disease when the dense diffuse breast involvement obscures the primary tumour (*Figure 2.52*).

Histological examination does not necessarily provide an answer. Simultaneous bilateral primary breast cancers and simultaneous primary and metastatic cancers may have the same histological features. In addition, a primary tumour of a particular histological type may give rise to metastases of another histological type.

The development of a second breast tumour in the contralateral breast following mastectomy occurs in about 10 per cent of cases (Stewart *et al.*, 1969; Egan, 1970). The occurrence of bilateral simultaneous carcinomas is uncommon in our experience. The possibility of its occurrence however should be borne in mind because it has an important bearing on the correct management of the patient.

Multiple irregular moderately dense lesions may be due to multifocal carcinoma, plasma cell mastitis or sclerosing adenosis.

The radiological features are similar to those previously described for solitary irregular lesions. All these conditions may commence as separate foci but later may become confluent.

Adenosis usually presents as multiple low density irregular lesions (*Figure 2.53*). It is usually bilateral but not necessarily of symmetrical distribution. The upper outer quadrant of the breast is most commonly affected.

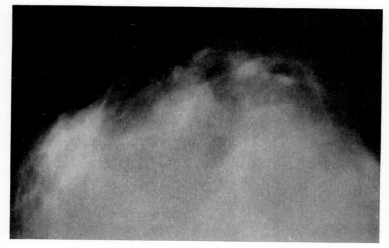

Figure 2.53. Diffuse adenosis. There are fluffy opacities throughout the breast

CO-EXISTING SMOOTH AND IRREGULAR LESIONS

Smooth and irregular lesions are found within the same breast in carcinoma with dysplasia, Schimmelbusch's mastopathy and fibro-adenosis with cysts.

Carcinoma with Dysplasia

The various breast dysplasias are common conditions. It is there-fore not surprising that carcinoma of the breast is frequently associ-ated with a variety of dysplasias such as fibroadenosis with cysts, fibroadenomas (*Figure 2.54*), secretory disease and Schimmelbusch's mastopathy (*Figure 2.55*).

Breast dysplasia may pre-dispose to carcinoma. Warren (1940) found an increased incidence of carcinoma in women with pre-existing breast disease. The incidence was 4·5 times greater for women of all ages and 11·7 times greater for women of less than 50 years of age.

Ingleby and Gershon-Cohen (1960) consider 'intra-ductal hyperplasia' to be the important pre-cancerous dysplasia. The term intraductal hyperplasia is synonymous with the terms epithelial hyperplasia and epitheliosis. Duct ectasia (secretory disease) is not considered as pre-disposing to malignancy. However enlarged ducts may be an indication of existing malignancy (Wolfe, 1967a) while en-largement due to epithelial hyperplasia would be an indication of a pre-malignant state. Scattered fine microcalcification may be present.

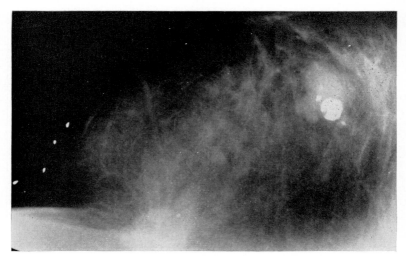

Figure 2.54. A spiculated carcinoma and a calcified fibroadenoma

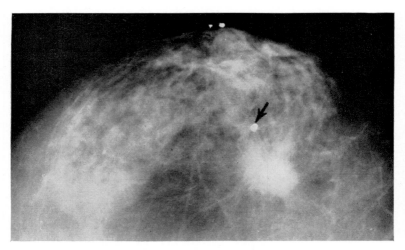

Figure 2.55. An impalpable spiculated carcinoma in a breast affected by Schimmel-busch's mastopathy. Whether the smooth calcified lesion is within the walls of a duct as in secretory disease or is calcified microcystic fat necrosis is not known

Leborgne (1967) has pointed out that the characteristic rounded calcification seen in secretory disease may be frequently confused with an entity which he calls 'microcystic calcified fat necrosis'.

These two conditions are often associated. In a series of 500 scirrhous carcinomas in older women 30 per cent of the cases showed calcified microcystic fat necrosis (*see Figure 2.55*). This might be a true association or a coincidence resulting from the age of the patients.

Schimmelbusch's Mastopathy

This mastopathy is said to occur when duct ectasia co-exists with other dysplasias such as fibroadenosis, cysts and fibroadenomas. The cysts and fibroadenomas and cystic dilatation of the ducts will give rise to smooth lesions. The irregular lesions may be due to sclerosing adenosis, plasma cell mastitis or abscess formation.

Fibroadenosis with Cysts

Adenosis and sclerosing adenosis are frequently associated with cyst formation so that irregular and smooth lesions may co-exist.

DIFFUSE LESIONS

The conditions giving rise to diffuse breast lesions are shown in Table 2.6.

TABLE 2.6

Diffuse Lesions

Dense opacities	*Moderately dense opacities*	*Low density opacities*
Carcinoma	Carcinoma	Adenosis
Reticulosis	Fibroadenosis with cysts and	Papillomatosis
Sarcoma	fibroadenomas	
Fibroadenosis	Plasma cell mastitis	
Infection		

Carcinoma

Diffuse involvement of the breast by carcinoma causes enlargement of the breast and usually a very marked increase in density. This increased density may be restricted to the glandular portion of the breast and then may be appreciated only by direct comparison with the opposite breast (*Figure 2.56*). In such cases the trabeculae and intra-glandular fat become obscured, but the subcutaneous fat remains transradiant.

Further progression will lead to haziness of the subcutaneous fat and thickening of Cooper's ligaments and the lymphatics together with generalized skin thickening (*Figure 2.57*). There will be hypervascularity and the original tumour may be only faintly visible or

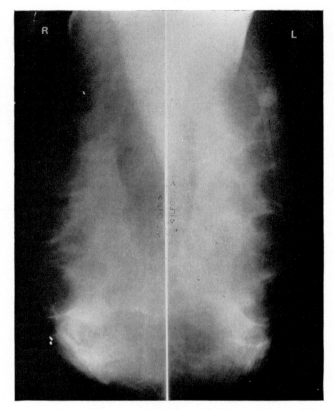

Figure 2.56. Axillary tail projections of right and left breast. There is diffuse malignant involvement of the left breast. Note increased density of the glandular tissue on the left side with hypervascularity. A notched lymph node is also seen on the left side. No involvement of subcutaneous fat

completely obscured. This appearance is found in the clinical entity known as 'inflammatory carcinoma' of the breast. However, it is stressed that this is a clinical diagnosis as the inflammatory element cannot be appreciated radiologically and diffuse infiltration without a clinical inflammatory response produces an identical mammographic appearance.

Reticulosis

The reticuloses can give a mammographic picture identical with that of diffuse carcinoma. Increase in density of the whole breast

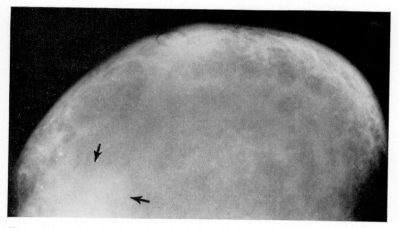

Figure 2.57. Diffuse malignancy of the breast with trabecular thickening, generalized oedema and skin thickening. The primary focus is arrowed. There is secretory disease or calcified microcystic fat necrosis also

occurs with prominence of trabeculae, lymphatics and suspensory ligaments. There is skin thickening and generalized oedema. The changes are due to involvement of the axillary nodes with consequent restricted lymph drainage.

Sarcoma

Although sarcoma usually presents as a smooth circumscribed dense breast lesion (*see* page 35) it may be diffuse when the mass is so large that it occupies the whole breast and when the pattern of involvement is one of diffuse infiltration (*see Figure 2.17*). These are, however, uncommon presentations.

Fibroadenosis

The changes in fibroadenosis may be mainly fibrous and in such cases with diffuse involvement the glandular portion of the breast assumes a dense homogeneous ground glass appearance (*Figure 2.58*). The changes are always bilateral but involvement is not necessarily equal on both sides. Trabeculae will be obscured and a few cysts or fibroadenomas may be faintly visible. The radiological features are similar to those found in immature breasts but are present in an older age group. In this type of breast a carcinoma may easily be obscured by the dense parenchyma. The skin and subcutaneous tissues are normal in the uncomplicated case and any change in these structures should arouse suspicion of malignancy.

71

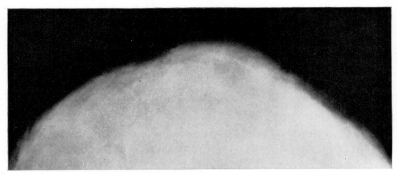

Figure 2.58. Dense fibrous changes of fibroadenosis in a woman aged 32 years. Compare with the normal immature breast (Figure 2.1)

Infection

Diffuse involvement of the breast with generalized oedema, hypervascularity, skin thickening and prominence of the subcutaneous reticulum may occur in bacterial mastitis and in particular tuberculous mastitis. It also occurs with acute abscess complicated by cellulitis. It may be impossible to distinguish between diffuse carcinoma and the oedematous type of tuberculosis. The clinical history will usually assist in differentiating carcinoma from acute abscess with cellulitis.

With moderately dense diffuse breast lesions a distinction will have to be made between carcinoma, fibroadenosis and plasma cell mastitis.

Carcinoma

When mammography is carried out early in the diffuse phase of carcinoma a generalized moderate increase in density is to be expected. Comparison with the opposite breast will assist in detecting such changes. The diffuse changes described above will be less obvious and the primary focus will usually be clearly visible.

Lobular carcinoma may be confined to a quadrant of the breast or be generalized and so give rise to diffuse changes (*see Figure 2.38*). These usually consist of multiple rounded opacities but some opacities may be partly or wholly indistinct in outline. The lesions are of moderate density and extreme difficulty may be experienced in distinguishing the condition from fibroadenosis with cysts and fibroadenomas. The existence of hypervascularity, oedema and skin thickening will assist in the differentiation.

Fibroadenosis with Cysts and Fibroadenomas

The appearances of fibroadenosis with cysts and fibroadenomas

72

have been previously described and illustrated (*see* pages 49, 50). Breast involvement is frequently diffuse and bilateral (*Figure 2.59*).

Plasma Cell Mastitis

Widespread involvement of the breast by plasma cell mastitis is uncommon but may occur. Multiple irregular densities will be superimposed on the changes of duct ectasia. The mastitic areas may become confluent and diffuse oedema and skin thickening may be apparent. The changes of duct ectasia will usually be bilateral but the plasma cell mastitis may be confined to one breast.

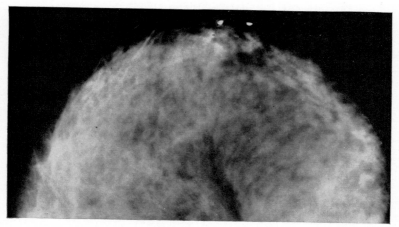

Figure 2.59. Diffuse fibroadenosis. There are numerous small rounded lesions which could be cysts, fibroadenomas or hyperplastic fibrotic nodules

Adenosis

Diffuse breast involvement occurs frequently giving rise to multiple fluffy opacities of ground glass density sometimes associated with hypervascularity (*Figure 2.53*). The changes are usually bilateral. Patchy areas of increased density will be found if sclerosing adenosis is present.

Papillomatosis

The lactiferous ducts may contain innumerable papillomas scattered throughout the duct system. In glandular breasts these may be very difficult to recognize being obscured by the parenchyma. In fatty and atrophic breasts they may be clearly seen giving a beaded appearance to the ducts. Close examination may reveal very small punctate calcific deposits in the line of the beaded ducts.

73

III—Disorders of Nipple and Skin. Calcification

NIPPLE LESIONS

There are two main clinical diagnostic problems, nipple retraction and Paget's disease of the nipple.

Nipple Retraction

The causes of nipple retraction as seen on mammograms are classified in Table 2.7. The appearances may be apparent rather than real.

TABLE 2.7

Nipple Retraction

Apparent retraction	Real retraction

Faulty radiographic positioning
Areolar oedema:
  inflammation
  diffuse carcinoma
	Congenital
	Acquired:
	  carcinoma
	  duct ectasia

Faulty positioning of the breast with failure to ensure that the nipple is in profile may give an erroneous impression of retraction. This is usually easily recognized. Areolar thickening as the result of oedema secondary to breast inflammation or diffuse carcinoma may give apparent inversion of the nipple due to a relative prominence of the areola. When the causative oedema subsides the nipple will be seen to be normal. True inversion of the nipple may be due to a congenital anomaly or may be acquired as a result of either carcinoma or duct ectasia.

Congenital retraction presents radiologically as a smooth rounded opacity in the sub-areolar region (*Figure 2.60*). Such retraction may be unilateral or bilateral. Patients are usually aware of this anomaly.

Acquired inversion is due to either carcinoma or duct ectasia. In carcinoma the inversion is usually unilateral but in duct ectasia it is frequently bilateral. However unilateral retraction may occur in duct ectasia and, because carcinoma may co-exist with duct ectasia, bilateral changes may be present. Rarely bilateral inversion may result from simultaneous bilateral carcinoma.

With malignant inversion a characteristic dense irregular lesion

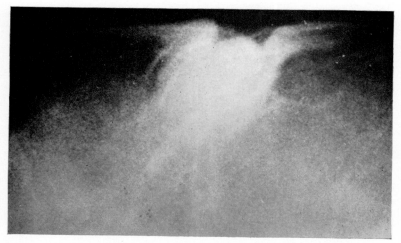

Figure 2.60. Congenital retraction of the nipple. The opacity is due to the nipple itself

(Reproduced from Evans and Gravelle (1969), by courtesy of the Editor, *X-ray Focus*.)

will be seen due to the tumour. It may be sub-areolar in position or may be situated some distance from the nipple when extension along the ducts to the nipple will be visible (*Figure 2.61*). The primary tumour may be palpable or impalpable.

Peri-ductal fibrosis is a common accompaniment of duct ectasia. When this is situated in the sub-areolar region it gives a conical opacity with the apex of the cone towards the nipple. It is practically always associated with nipple inversion. The mammographic appearances will be characteristic with dilated ducts and a sub-areolar conical opacity. Frequently there is associated smooth rounded calcification of burnt-out secretory disease (*Figure 2.62*).

When clinical inversion occurs in the absence of a palpable mass, mammography is an important investigation because it may demon-

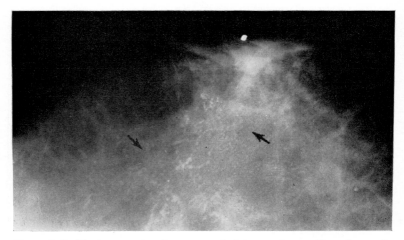

Figure 2.61. Nipple retraction due to an underlying carcinoma. Note the areolar thickening, hypervascularity and characteristic malignant microcalcification. Punctate and elongated types of calcification are present

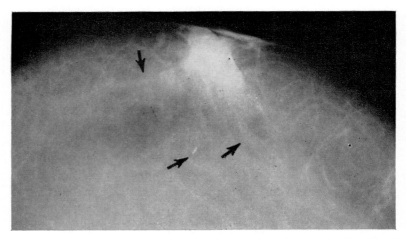

Figure 2.62. Duct ectasia with sub-areolar fibrosis and nipple retraction. The dilated ducts can be seen deep to the retracted nipple. The calcification of secretory disease is also present

strate an impalpable carcinoma or allay the fears of the clinician by demonstrating a benign cause for the retraction.

Paget's Disease of the Nipple

Clinically this condition may be difficult to differentiate from simple eczema of the nipple. Paget's disease presents as an eczema-like lesion of the nipple eventually progressing to erosion and destruction. In the early stages the underlying intra-duct carcinoma is impalpable.

Mammography may show characteristic microcalcification indicating intra-duct carcinoma which may be either localized in the sub-areolar region or widespread (*Figure 2.63*). Alternatively a

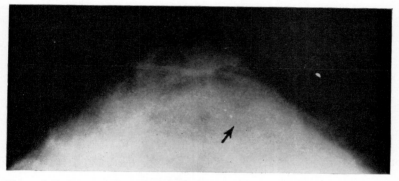

Figure 2.63. Punctate microcalcification of intra-duct carcinoma associated with Paget's disease of the nipple

small spiculated lesion may be seen denoting an invasive carcinoma. If there is no radiological evidence of malignancy, in the absence of a palpable lesion further management should include repeated mammography at 6-monthly intervals. In this way an early indication of malignant change may be obtained.

SKIN LESIONS

Dermal lesions of the breast may be localized or ulcerated. They can present as localized or generalized skin thickening. The causes of these changes are shown in Table 2.8. In order to be able to determine radiologically that a skin lesion is present the x-ray beam will have to pass through the lesion tangentially. Otherwise localized rounded skin lesions could in such circumstances appear to be situated within the breast. There will be no problem when generalized skin thickening is present but localized thickening and ulceration could be overlooked.

TABLE 2.8

Skin Lesions

Localized and rounded	Ulceration	Skin thickening
Cysts—sebaceous, apocrine Neoplasm—benign: warts, naevi, etc malignant: metastases apocrine carcinoma	Carcinoma Sarcoma Giant fibroadenoma Mammillary fistula Tuberculosis	Localized: carcinoma plasma cell mastitis abscess trauma: contusion biopsy Generalized: carcinoma infection lymphoma scleroderma

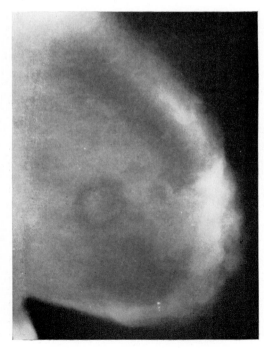

Figure 2.64. Malignant skin nodules from breast carcinoma. There is associated skin thickening. Note how one of the nodules appears to be within the breast

(Reproduced from Evans and Gravelle (1969), by courtesy of the Editor, *X-ray Focus*.)

Sebaceous and apocrine cysts will present with smooth, rounded opacities indistinguishable from each other. Apocrine cysts occur frequently in the axillary regions because the apocrine glands are common in this situation. Skin naevi will appear flatter than cysts.

Malignant secondary deposits, especially of breast origin, may be associated with skin thickening (*Figure 2.64*). Apocrine carcinoma will usually be axillary in position and will present as a dense circumscribed lesion often with associated skin thickening.

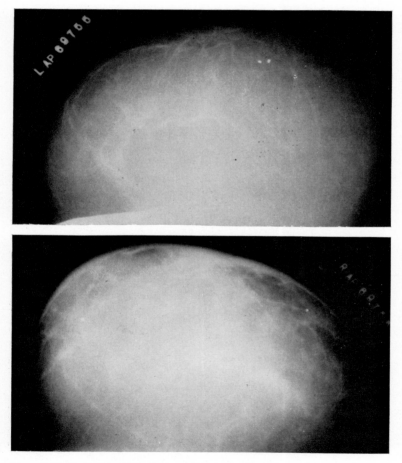

Figure 2.65. Early skin thickening may be more easily recognized by comparing the two breasts

Mammary carcinoma and sarcoma may give rise to ulceration of the overlying skin. The underlying breast abnormality will be obvious. Giant fibroadenoma may cause ulceration due to the marked stretching of the skin in this condition. In mammillary fistula the underlying duct ectasia, plasma cell mastitis and abscess will be evident but no specific changes will be present in tuberculosis. Localized and generalized skin thickening can be clearly seen in the mammograms and the changes may be obvious even though clinically there is no indication of skin abnormality. By comparing mammograms of both breasts the earliest changes will be easily recognized (*Figure 2.65*).

Localized skin thickening will be associated with the features of the underlying lesion such as carcinoma (*see Figure 2.45*), plasma cell mastitis (*see Figure 2.46*) and abscess (*see Figure 2.22*). The contused breast may be normal apart from the skin thickening but if the trauma is due to biopsy there will usually be an underlying breast abnormality which necessitated biopsy. Aspiration biopsy, drill biopsy (*Figure 2.66*) and operative biopsy will cause localized skin thickening.

If lead markers are used and attached by Sellotape, care should be taken that there is no wrinkling of the skin because localized skin thickening may then be simulated. In addition, it should be remembered that the skin of the lower half of the breast on the medio-lateral projection may appear thickened as a result of wrinkling of the skin due to faulty positioning. Comparison of the two medio-lateral projections will indicate the true state of affairs. This is important be-

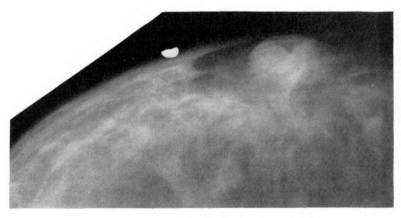

Figure 2.66. Localized skin thickening due to drill biopsy

(Reproduced from Evans and Gravelle (1969), by courtesy of the Editor, *X-ray Focus*.

cause early generalized thickening may be noticed first over the lower half of the breast.

With generalized thickening of the skin the aetiological factor may be apparent (*see Figure 2.57*) or obscured by the associated marked density of the breast tissue, as for instance with diffuse carcinoma (*see Figure 2.52*). A similar appearance occurs in the oedematous type of tuberculosis of the breast. Enlarged axillary nodes in lymphoma may produce generalized skin thickening and a diffuse opacity in the breast as a result of lymphatic obstruction.

LACTIFEROUS DUCT LESIONS

Duct lesions frequently give rise to nipple discharge but this symptom may also develop in fibroadenosis with cysts. The discharge may be the only symptom or there may be a palpable mass. The causes of nipple discharge are given in Table 2.9.

TABLE 2.9

Causes of Nipple Discharge

---

1. Fibroadenosis
2. Duct ectasia
3. Granuloma
4. Abscess
5. Lactation:
    (*a*) Normal involution
    (*b*) Galactocoele
    (*c*) Lactating fibroadenoma
6. Epithelial hyperplasia
7. Papillary tumour:
    (*a*) Papilloma
    (*b*) Endoductal fibroadenoma
8. Carcinoma:
    (*a*) Non-infiltrative papilliferous intra-duct carcinoma
    (*b*) Intra-duct carcinoma
    (*c*) Paget's disease of the nipple
    (*d*) Infiltrating carcinoma

Clinical assessment and examination of the discharge both by direct inspection and microscopy are important. A bacteriological examination may be necessary and the discharge should always be tested for the presence of blood. As well as these procedures, mammography alone and following contrast examination of the ducts, provides valuable additional information. The diagnosis may be established by these radiological methods and the clinical diagnosis thus confirmed or refuted. Impalpable lesions may be demonstrated and accurate localization of the underlying pathology may be achieved. Having demonstrated the location, nature and extent of the disease process a rational approach to therapy is obtained.

The various types of nipple discharge are commonly associated with specific disorders. For example, a clear serous discharge is frequently due to fibroadenosis with cysts but may also occur in duct ectasia and occasionally in carcinoma and papilloma. Papilloma is undoubtedly the commonest cause of blood-stained nipple discharge but this may occur with carcinoma, duct ectasia, granuloma, abscess, epithelial hyperplasia and in the later stages of pregnancy and during lactation.

A black, brownish or greenish discharge may be due to altered blood but is also commonly associated with the cysts of fibroadenosis. A purulent discharge is indicative of a breast abscess which may or may not be associated with plasma cell mastitis. Milky discharge is usually the result of previous lactation and can sometimes be expressed after lactation has ceased. It may also be due to a galactocoele, a lactating fibroadenoma or secretory disease.

The important fact to remember is that a malignant lesion may be present with any type of discharge and does not necessarily cause blood-staining of the discharge. Equally important—other lesions can give rise to a blood-stained nipple discharge but naturally in the presence of such a discharge a thorough search for a malignant lesion must be undertaken.

Mammography usually shows enlargement of the lactiferous ducts. These may be clearly visible on the radiograph but injection of the discharging duct with contrast medium may be necessary in order to demonstrate the enlargement. The greater the amount of fat within the breast, the more easily will the ducts be seen. Mammographic changes of associated lesions may be present—for example, subareolar fibrosis and plasma cell mastitis. Different types of microcalcification will give an indication of the underlying process.

The causes of duct enlargement are given in Table 2.10. The carci-

TABLE 2.10

Causes of Enlargement of Lactiferous Ducts

1. Duct ectasia
2. Papillomatosis
3. Granuloma
4. Epithelial hyperplasia
5. Carcinoma:
   (*a*) Intra-ductal
      (*i*) Papilliferous
      (*ii*) Non-papilliferous
   (*b*) Invasive

noma may be entirely intra-ductal and papilliferous or non-papilliferous. Alternatively the malignancy may be invasive. The enlargement in such cases may be the result of intra-ductal growth or non-specific enlargement due to blockage of the duct.

On plain radiography duct ectasia may show cystic dilatation confined to one portion of a single duct or many ducts may show the anomaly. The mammographic appearances may be indistinguishable from those of solitary or multiple cysts in such cases. A whole duct may be dilated giving a smooth cylindrical tortuous opacity. This change is easily recognizable but more commonly several ducts are involved in the process (*Figure 2.67*). The changes of sub-areolar

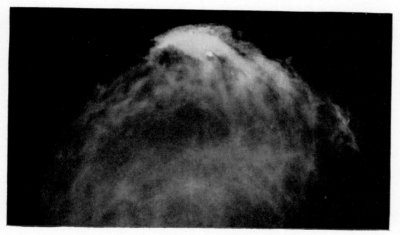

Figure 2.67. Duct ectasia. Numerous dilated ducts are present

fibrosis (*see Figure 2.62*) and plasma cell mastitis (*see Figure 2.46*) may be present. Occasionally the enlarged ducts will be seen as transradiant structures (*Figure 2.68*) rather than as opacities. Leborgne (1953) considered this appearance to be due to air filling of the ducts but as the condition is associated, in our experience, with a milky nipple discharge it is probably due to the high fat content of the duct secretions. Confirmation of this view has been obtained after injection of the affected ducts (*Figure 2.68*). No air bubbles are present in the contrast-filled duct; being fluid, the duct contents have mixed with the contrast medium.

Patients who present with nipple discharge with or without an associated palpable lesion should have mammography carried out initially. If on inspection of these mammograms there is no evidence

83

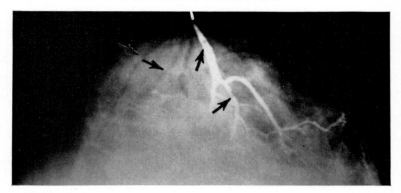

Figure 2.68. Several dilated transradiant ducts are seen. This is due to the high fat level of the duct contents. Contrast examination confirms the dilatation and shows inspissated secretions also

of malignancy then contrast examination is indicated even though there may be plain film evidence of duct ectasia or fibroadenosis.

Contrast examination may confirm the original plain film diagnosis—as for example in fibroadenosis with cysts (*Figure 2.69*). Alternatively it may show two unsuspected duct disorders co-existing (*Figures 2.67* and *2.70*). On mammography a diagnosis of duct ectasia was made in this patient who presented with blood-stained nipple discharge. Contrast examination confirmed the duct ectasia but also showed a papilloma to be present. A papilloma may be simulated by air bubble, inspissated secretion, granuloma, blood clot or intraductal fibroadenoma. If the filling defect on contrast examination is

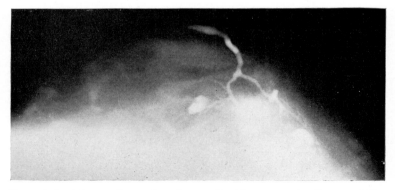

Figure 2.69. A few small cysts have been outlined by contrast in this case of fibroadenosis

84

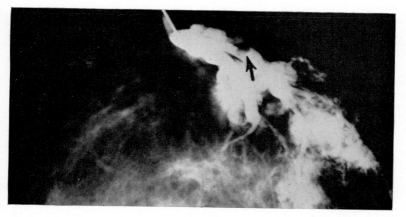

Figure 2.70. Same case as in Figure 2.67. The duct ectasia is confirmed but a smooth lobulated papilloma is also shown to be present

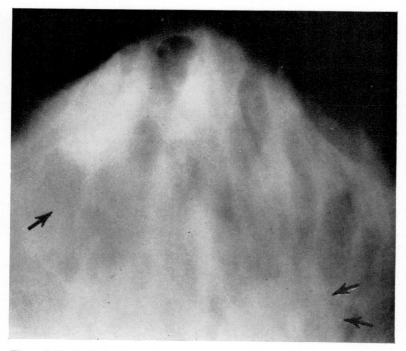

Figure 2.71. Epithelial hyperplasia. There is diffuse adenosis and very faint fine scattered calcification is present. There is a cyst deep in the breast also

85

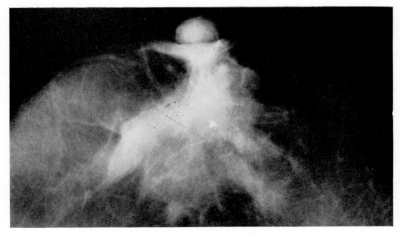

Figure 2.72. Non-infiltrative papilliferous intra-duct carcinoma. The involved ducts are enormously dilated and fine punctate microcalcification is present

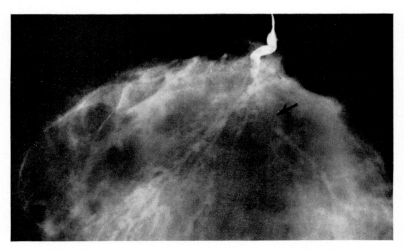

Figure 2.73. Contrast examination showing multiple filling defects in the ducts due to papilliferous intra-duct carcinoma. An irregular stricture is also shown thus demonstrating an unsuspected and impalpable carcinoma

86

single, discrete and slightly polypoid it is likely to be a papilloma. A more irregular multi-focal lesion is likely to be due to inspissated secretion or blood clot. Multiple papillomas may also occur.

Epithelial hyperplasia may give enlargement of the lactiferous ducts but is usually recognized on account of the scattered fine punctate microcalcification which may be present (*Figure 2.71*). The condition is pre-cancerous and may lead to intra-ductal carcinoma.

Non-infiltrative papilliferous intra-duct carcinoma usually gives rise to marked enlargement of the involved ducts (*Figures 2.10* and *2.72*). The enlarged ducts are smooth and may contain flecks of calcification. There is usually hypervascularity. Any associated irregularity of the margins of the enlarged ducts should raise the suspicion that invasion has occurred. If the ducts are not obviously enlarged contrast examination will be necessary to diagnose the condition (*Figure 2.73*). A blood-stained discharge due to a carcinoma may be present in patients without a palpable mass and with normal mammographic findings. Contrast examination in such patients may reveal an irregular stricture due to an unsuspected carcinoma (*Figure 2.73*).

Non-papilliferous intra-duct carcinoma usually shows characteristic microcalcification which may or may not be associated with dilated ducts (*Figure 2.74*).

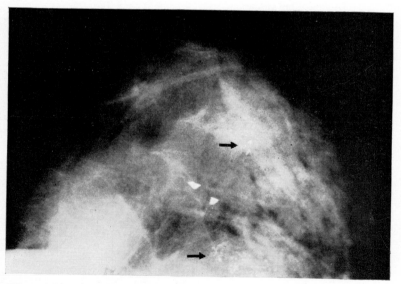

Figure 2.74. Characteristic microcalcification in intra-duct carcinoma. Some is punctate and some elongated but all is irregular

CALCIFICATION

The presence of calcification on a mammogram is of great importance diagnostically as it is one of the direct radiographic signs of malignancy and benign disease. In the vast majority of cases it will enable the radiologist to make a firm diagnosis of the nature of the breast disease present. It must be borne in mind however that more than one disease process may co-exist and that the microcalcification may be an indication of the least significant lesion present. In addition although florid calcific changes are invariably pathognomonic of the underlying disease, calcification may be present in such small amount that a definite radiological diagnosis cannot be made.

Calcification of the media of breast arteries occurs normally in elderly patients (*see Figure 2.7*). It may also be seen in chronic renal failure as a feature of metastatic calcification. Apart from these arterial changes calcification patterns are usually characteristic of either malignant or benign breast disease. The various changes are given in Tables 2.11 and 2.12.

TABLE 2.11	TABLE 2.12
Calcification in Malignant Disease	*Calcification in Benign Disease*

1. Fine and irregular:
    Punctate or granular
    Elongated—straight or curved
    Filigree or serpiginous
	1. Coarse and smooth
	    Peripheral in position
	    Central in position
	    Rounded, ovoid, lobulated or ring-like
	    Elongated, tubular and branched
	    Bizarre

2. Coarse and irregular:
    Flake-like
	2. Fine and smooth:
	    Punctate—localized or scattered
	    Elongated—localized or scattered
	    Eggshell

3. Rarely coarse and smooth	

The use of fine grain industrial type film and slight over-exposure of the mammogram will ensure that microcalcification will be visible in the maximum number of cases. This should be shown in 30–40 per cent of instances of malignant disease and to a lesser extent in benign conditions. The diagnostic features depend on the appearance and distribution of the calcifications.

In Malignant Disease

In the majority of cases in malignant disease, microcalcification will have irregular margins although it may be necessary at times to use a magnifying glass to appreciate this. As well as being irregular in outline the particles will usually be small in size.

The malignant calcifications may be punctate or granular in character (*Figures 2.61* and *2.74*). Elongated particles are frequently seen and these may be curved or straight. Such particles have been likened to the broken ends of needles (*Figures 2.61* and *2.74*). Less commonly the calcification is serpiginous or gives rise to a fine filigree pattern (*Figure 2.75*).

Occasionally coarse calcification occurs in malignant disease. Even in cases of intra-duct carcinoma some of the calcific particles are much larger in size than the majority. In mucoid carcinoma and cystosarcoma phylloides coarse flake-like calcification may be seen. Even though the calcification is coarse in these cases it is always irregular in outline (*see Figure 2.13*). Very rarely malignant lesions may contain smooth coarse calcification. This may occur on original presentation or following radiotherapy (*Figure 2.76*).

The distribution of the calcification is characteristic. In intra-duct or 'comedo-carcinoma' the calcification occurs along the lines of the lactiferous ducts and enlargement of the ducts may not be visible. In such cases there is a polarity of the particles but in many instances there may be no polarity and the granules are scattered apparently at random (*see Figures 2.61* and *2.74*). The changes may be localized to a small area of the breast or widespread. When microcalcification is the only indication of malignancy the lesion may be impalpable even in the presence of extensive disease. The calcification may be localized within a small dense irregular mass indicating an invasive

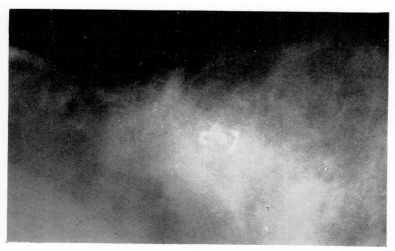

Figure 2.75. Serpiginous calcification in carcinoma

89

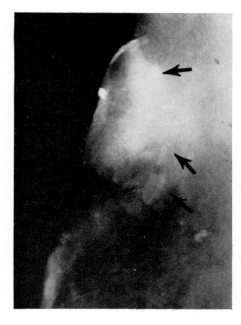

Figure 2.76. Coarse smooth calcification which developed in the carcinoma following radiotherapy

scirrhous carcinoma (*Figure 2.77*). Less commonly microcalcification occurs within a circumscribed carcinoma. The calcification may be partly distributed within an obvious carcinoma and partly at a distance from the visible mass (*see Figure 2.42*). Presumably in such cases the original intra-duct carcinoma has become invasive at the site of the mass.

Calcific changes are seen in all kinds of breast carcinoma. They occur mainly in necrotic areas especially in intra-duct carcinoma but may also occur in viable malignant tissue within and outside the ducts.

In Benign Disease

Calcification in benign breast disease has a smooth outline irrespective of whether it is coarse or fine in type. In the majority of cases such calcification is of a coarse nature and is much larger than that usually found in malignant disease.

The calcification may be situated in the periphery of the lesion as in some fibroadenomas (*see Figure 2.35*) or cysts (*see Figure 2.20*). A peripheral distribution is also seen in fat necrosis and secretory disease (*see Figure 2.48*). Amorphous dense central calcification is

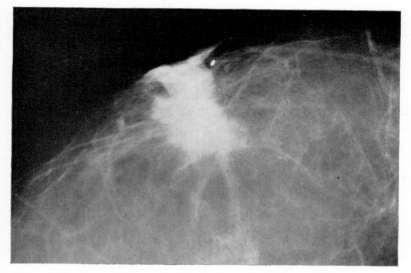

Figure 2.77. Microcalcification within a small scirrhous carcinoma causing retraction of the nipple

common in fibroadenomas (*see Figure 2.11*) and may also occur in fat necrosis. The calcifications may be rounded, ovoid or lobulated in shape usually conforming to the shape of the underlying lesion. They may also be ring-like. Elongated coarse tubular calcification, sometimes branching, is seen in the line of the ducts in secretory disease (*see Figure 2.48*). Bizarre coral-like coarse calcification may be seen in fibroadenomas.

When the calcification is fine and smooth it may exhibit the so-called 'eggshell calcification' (*see Figure 2.20*). The type is not pathognomonic of cysts as it may be found in cystic fat necrosis (Leborgne, 1967) and in haematomas.

A difficult diagnostic problem arises when benign calcification is of the fine type. It may be punctate or elongated and both forms may occur together. When this is so the problem is one of distinction between malignancy and benign disease because the radiographic appearances may be very similar and even indistinguishable in such cases. These types of calcification may be found in sclerosing adenosis, epithelial hyperplasia and papillomas. Frequently in sclerosing adenosis and epithelial hyperplasia the calcifications are scattered throughout the breast and are usually bilateral in distribution. Occasionally however the calcified particles are few in number and

91

localized to one small area of the breast. Papillomas may give identical appearances and an attempt has to be made to distinguish the benign conditions from a small intra-duct carcinoma. The papilloma will usually give rise to blood-stained nipple discharge and may thus be diagnosed by contrast examination of the discharging duct.

Localized calcification due to epithelial hyperplasia or sclerosing adenosis may be associated with scattered fine calcification and this may help the radiologist to come to a decision. If the calcification is smooth on examination with a magnifying glass this will also indicate a benign lesion. There will always be some doubt in these cases as to the nature of the underlying pathology particularly as epithelial hyperplasia is a pre-cancerous condition. Intra-duct carcinoma may also occur in a breast displaying the changes of epithelial hyperplasia so that biopsy of the suspicious area will be indicated. As the lesion will be impalpable radiographic control of the biopsy will be necessary. The quadrant containing the calcification will already have been located from mammography. A specimen of breast tissue should immediately be radiographed to confirm that the suspicious area of calcification has been removed from the breast. This can be carried out before closure of the biopsy wound. The area of the specimen containing the calcification can be further pin-pointed by inserting

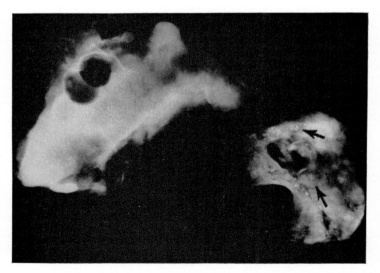

Figure 2.78. Radiograph of mounted specimens showing localization of microcalcification

(Reproduced by courtesy of Dr. W. Foort.)

92

needles in appropriate positions according to the findings on radiography. The specimen can then be divided and again the mounted blocks radiographed in order to confirm the presence and position of the calcification within the various portions of the breast specimen (*Figure 2.78*).

Chapter 3

Mammography—Evaluation and Indications

DIFFICULTIES IN INTERPRETATION

It is essential for the interpretation of mammograms to obtain films of good quality. Correct exposure is a vital factor in producing films of good contrast so that malignant microcalcification and the margins of lesions can be demonstrated. Inadequate positioning may result in a significant lesion not being projected on to the film. Lesions deep within the breast, especially in the inner half, the infra-clavicular region and also in the axillary tail area, are difficult to demonstrate well. The axillary tail view will however allow adequate visualization of this area. These difficulties in positioning are exaggerated in small breasts; if the glandular tissue in such breasts is dense then a carcinoma which is obvious clinically may be easily obscured on the mammogram. The denser the breast tissue the more difficult the demonstration of a lesion within that breast becomes. Conversely the greater the amount of fat within the breast the easier the visualization of a breast lesion. Even small carcinomas of 0·5 cm diameter may be clearly seen in fatty atrophic breasts.

As mentioned in the preceding chapter difficulties in interpretation of microcalcification arise in cases in which there is fine sparse localized calcification. In such cases differentiation between intra-duct carcinoma, epithelial hyperplasia and sclerosing adenosis may not be possible and excision biopsy is indicated.

The main problem will usually arise in the differentiation of smooth circumscribed lesions. The distinction between a cyst and a fibro-adenoma may not always be possible but this is not clinically important. However, distinguishing these lesions from a circumscribed carcinoma or sarcoma is vital. The malignant lesion will usually be very dense and careful examination of its margins may show an area of irregularity which, in association with hypervascularity, trabecular

94

distortion and oedema, will indicate the true nature of the lesion. Unfortunately some carcinomas show only moderate or even low radiodensity, while some benign cysts and fibroadenomas may present opacities of considerable density. Again small irregularities of outline, the presence of microcalcification and association of the secondary signs of malignancy will be important features. The application of Leborgne's law will assist the radiologist in arriving at the correct diagnosis. Another problem is the differentiation of giant fibroadenomas from cystosarcoma phylloides. This may be impossible but if coarse irregular calcification is present then this is an indication of cystosarcoma or sarcomatous degeneration.

The association of a small circumscribed moderately dense carcinoma with a cystic breast dysplasia will tax the diagnostic abilities of the radiologist. Differentiation of these lesions may not be possible.

Occasionally irregular lesions such as plasma cell mastitis and sclerosing adenosis may cause difficulty in interpretation. The association of plasma cell mastitis with duct ectasia and its frequent clinical presentation with considerable pain in the involved area are additional pointers to the correct diagnosis. Sclerosing adenosis may be clinically and radiologically indistinguishable from carcinoma. In such cases the radiologist should make it quite clear that there is doubt as to the nature of the lesion and that biopsy is indicated.

EVALUATION

The value of mammography depends on its accuracy both in demonstrating the various breast diseases and in distinguishing between malignant and benign conditions. Numerous studies of the accuracy of the method have been reported. The results of some of these studies are shown in Table 3.1.

Our accuracy rates have been previously reported (Stewart *et al.*,

TABLE 3.1

Overall Accuracy in Mammographic Diagnosis

	No. of lesions	*Accuracy rate*
Egan (1964)	1,217	94·6%
Samuel and Young (1964)	450	90%
Wolfe (1964)	674	89%
Gershon-Cohen and Forman (1964)	500	90%
Friedman *et al.* (1966)	776	88%

All lesions histologically confirmed.

1969). The overall accuracy in 623 lesions confirmed by biopsy was 88 per cent. Of 302 carcinomas the overall mammographic accuracy was 93 per cent. When these 302 malignant lesions were divided into advanced inoperable cases and operable cases then the accuracy for the 136 advanced carcinomas was 98 per cent and for the 166 operable carcinomas, 89 per cent.

A more recent evaluation of our mammographic diagnostic results in 1,156 cases showed an accuracy of 87 per cent in the diagnosis of malignant disease and of 97 per cent in benign disease.

The technique therefore provides an accurate means of diagnosing breast lesions. It is frequently more accurate than clinical diagnosis, the accuracy of which varies in reported cases from 75 per cent (Sandison, 1958) to 88 per cent (Stewart et al., 1969). Even though this is lower than the mammographic accuracy rate, however, the important feature is that some tumours will have definite clinical features of malignancy when mammographically they may appear benign or may not even be visible. Conversely some lesions obviously malignant on mammography may clinically appear to be benign or may be impalpable. Consequently the two methods of examination are complementary procedures. By using both methods a diagnostic accuracy rate of the order of 97 per cent may be expected in breast malignancy (Stewart et al., 1969).

Mammography therefore increases the pre-operative diagnostic accuracy. An unsuspected lesion is frequently found in the opposite breast even when symptoms or clinical abnormality are restricted to one breast. In addition in clinically normal or benign cases the technique can give further reassurance by confirming the clinical impression.

Serial examination by mammography will enable an objective assessment to be made of the response of malignant lesions to palliative therapy. These radiographs then present a unique record, useful for review and subsequent management. Similarly the method is of use in management of the contralateral breast following mastectomy for carcinoma where there is an increased incidence of a second malignancy in the remaining breast. In a reported series (Stewart et al., 1969) of contralateral breast examinations in 384 patients over a period of 5 years, 39 carcinomas were found, an incidence of 10·1 per cent. Of these 39 cancers, 11 were unsuspected clinically.

Egan (1970) and Ingleby and Gershon-Cohen (1960) are of the opinion that mammography is of value in assessing the prognosis in breast cancer. They maintain that the type of contour of the malignant lesion as shown on the mammogram is an indication of its malignancy and consequently of the prognosis. It is maintained that tumours with irregular outlines have a significantly higher mortality than those with a circumscribed outline.

There is no doubt that mammography gives an accurate indication of the morphology of breast tumours. However it is the histological features that are important in prognosis and these cannot be shown in mammograms. In addition the morphological type is not restricted to any particular histological type. Even when an impalpable intra-duct carcinoma is shown radiologically as a result of characteristic microcalcification and in the absence of mammographic evidence of invasion, lymph gland metastases may be present.

Periodic clinical examination of the breast by a skilled clinician and the technique of self palpation are not in themselves adequate methods for the early detection of breast cancer. Radiographic techniques may assist considerably in reaching an early diagnosis of this condition.

Clinically Undiagnosed Breast Cancer

Unrecognized breast cancers are either mis-diagnosed palpable tumours or are impalpable. Cases fall into two main categories as shown in Table 3.2.

TABLE 3.2

Early Radiological Detection of Clinically Undiagnosed Breast Cancer

Palpable lesions present	*No lesion palpable*
Solitary lesion, clinically benign Multiple lesions. No dominant lesion	Vague breast symptoms only Asymptomatic

Presence of Palpable Lesions

Solitary.—In the first group palpable lesions are present. A solitary lesion may be present which has benign features on clinical examination. Mammography is of great value in these cases and contrast examination of the ducts can contribute additional useful information. Radiological examination may help in three ways:

(1) It may show conclusively that the lesion is malignant.

(2) The mammogram may confirm that the palpable lesion is benign in nature but that there is also a malignant lesion elsewhere in the breast.

(3) Alternatively it may show a carcinoma in the contralateral breast or even bilateral carcinomas.

Multiple.—The second sub-group consist of cases in which there are multiple palpable lesions, usually bilateral in distribution. Unsuspected malignancies may occur in such lumpy breasts in the absence of a dominant lesion. Mammography can distinguish between benign and malignant lesions in such cases and lead to earlier diagnosis of the malignancy (*see Figure 2.55*).

Absence of Palpable Lesions

Vague symptoms.—In the second main group the patient has no palpable lesion but may have vague breast symptoms such as discomfort, an unusual pain or a discharge or there may be an eczematous lesion of the nipple. Mammography is essential in such cases and contrast examination of the ducts may be indicated as well. An impalpable carcinoma may be shown radiographically in the following circumstances:

(1) intra-duct carcinoma showing pathognomonic microcalcification only (*see Figure 2.74*);

(2) Paget's disease of the nipple, when characteristic microcalcification of intra-duct carcinoma or a small spiculated carcinoma may be shown (*see Figure 2.63*);

(3) when the breast is large and the tumour small. Even a 5-mm tumour is readily shown in a large fatty breast since here radiographic contrast is enhanced.

When there is nipple discharge of whatever type, contrast examination of the ducts is indicated as an underlying carcinoma may be demonstrated. *Figure 2.73* shows the mammogram (with duct injection) of a young woman with a blood-stained nipple discharge with no palpable lesion in the breast. Clinically she was thought to have a papilloma but contrast examination showed multiple filling defects which were interpreted as being papilliferous intra-duct carcinoma and one area was shown to be invasive.

Asymptomatic.—The next and final group consists of those patients whose tumours are both without symptoms and impalpable. These can be discovered only by screening programmes. We have recently compared the accuracy of clinical examination and mammography in 891 women. Of these, 414 women had symptoms of breast disease and 477 were without breast symptoms. Clinical information was available to the radiologist. In the asymptomatic group no malignant disease was encountered. No malignancy was suspected on clinical examination but one case was suspected of malignancy on mammography; however, this was disproved.

Relative Diagnostic Accuracy

Of the 414 patients in the symptomatic group, 297 had benign

TABLE 3.3

	All cases (414)	Proven benign (145)	Malignant (77)	Malignant (operable) (59)	Malignant (inoperable) (18)
Clinical examination	88%	81%	82%	76%	100%
Mammography	95%	95%	85%	80%	100%

lesions (145 confirmed histologically and 152 were regarded as benign on follow-up examination), 40 patients were considered to be normal and 77 had malignant lesions (69 confirmed histologically and 8 with clinically obvious malignancy). The relative diagnostic accuracy of clinical and mammographic examination in the symptomatic group is shown in Table 3.3. The false negatives were 18 per cent for clinical examination and 15 per cent for mammography. The false positives were 19 per cent for clinical examination and 5 per cent for mammography.

Table 3.4 shows the combined results in the 77 malignancies referred to above. Clinical and radiographic examinations are complementary. Neither method should be used in isolation in the screening of women for breast cancer. An important New York study compared the mortality from breast cancer in women who had regular annual screening by clinical examination and mammography with that of those who received normal medical care (Strax et al., 1967/68/69; Venet et al., 1969). Although the final evaluation must await assessment of mortality, it is already apparent that cases of breast cancer discovered in the screened group have a lower incidence of lymphatic involvement than those arising in the controls.

TABLE 3.4

Clinical examination alone	82%
Mammography alone	85%
Clinical examination and mammography	90%

INDICATIONS

Following this consideration of the value of mammography it is evident that the indications for mammography may be summarized as follows:

Confirmation of the Clinical Diagnosis

Even if the breast lesion is obviously malignant clinically, mammographic examination will enable the radiologist to extend his interpretative experience and the radiographer to practise the art of mammography. Occasionally, even in these cases, the mammogram will disprove the clinical diagnosis so that biopsy will be indicated rather than the more drastic surgical treatment.

Diagnostic Aid in Clinically Difficult or Doubtful Cases

The technique is of value in breast dysplasias, large fatty breasts, Paget's disease of the nipple without a palpable lump and also in gynaecomastia.

Examination of Cases Clinically Unsuspected of Breast Carcinoma

In the presence of vague breast symptoms or nipple discharge the examination may indicate the presence of a malignant lesion or reassure the clinician as to the benign nature of the underlying breast disease. Pre-operative mammography will help to exclude unsuspected carcinomas in the contralateral breast. It may also be useful in the demonstration of a primary malignant focus in the presence of metastases.

Breast Biopsy

The examination will be the only indication of the correct biopsy site in impalpable carcinomas. It may also be used to confirm that a suspicious area has been removed at biopsy either by examination of the breast following biopsy or more conveniently by radiography of the biopsy specimen. In addition mammography may indicate that a lesion of the breast is definitely malignant so that mastectomy may be planned rather than biopsy. However, although a benign lesion may be demonstrated, biopsy should still be encouraged as in a small percentage of cases mammography will be inaccurate.

Long Term Management

The technique is useful in the periodic examination of the contralateral breast following mastectomy for carcinoma. It is also useful in the follow-up of a lesion that has not been subjected to surgery whether such a lesion is benign or malignant. Again, it is an excellent method for assessment of the effect of palliative radiotherapy or chemotherapy on an inoperable tumour.

Certainly soft tissue radiographic examination of the breast is a valuable complementary procedure in the diagnosis and management of breast diseases.

100

REFERENCES

Mammography

Berger, S. M. and Gershon-Cohen, J. (1962). Mammography of breast sarcoma. *American Journal of Roentgenology*, **87**, 76–81.

Bjørn-Hansen, R. (1965). Contrast mammography. *British Journal of Radiology*, **38**, 947–951.

Black, J. W. and Young, G. B. (1965). A radiological and pathological study of the incidence of calcification in diseases of the breast and neoplasms of other tissues. *British Journal of Radiology*, **38**, 596–598.

Dobretsberger, W. (1962). Isodensography. *X-Ray Bulletin*, **4**, 12–15.

— (1967). Fluidography of the female breast. *Electromedica*, **4**, 12–15.

Egan, R. L. (1960). Experience with mammography in a tumour institution: evaluation of 1,000 studies. *Radiology*, **75**, 894–900.

— (1964). *Mammography*. Springfield, Ill.; Thomas.

— (1968). *Technologist Guide to Mammography*. Baltimore; Williams and Wilkins.

— (1970). Mammography and breast diseases. Section 19, *Golden's Diagnostic Radiology*. Baltimore; Williams and Wilkins.

Evans, K. T. and Gravelle, I. H. (1969). Mammography Symposium—1. An important ancillary method of investigation. *X-ray Focus*, **9**, 3–10.

Foote, F. W. Jr. and Stewart, F. W. (1941). Lobular carcinoma in situ. *American Journal of Pathology*, **17**, 491–496.

Friedman, A. K., Askovitz, S. I., Berger, S. M., Dodd, G. D., Fisher, M. S., Lapayowker, M. S., Moore, J. P., Parlee, D. E., Stein, G. N. and Pendergrass, E. P. (1966). A co-operative evaluation of mammography in seven teaching hospitals. *Radiology*, **86**, 886–891.

Furnival, Isobel, G., Stewart, Helen, J., Weddell, J. M., Dovey, P., Gravelle, I. H., Evans, K. T. and Forrest, A. P. M. (1970). Accuracy of screening methods for the diagnosis of breast disease. *British Medical Journal*, **4**, 461–463.

Gershon-Cohen, J. (1970). *Modern Trends in Diagnostic Radiology—4*, Chapter 6. Ed. by J. W. McLaren. London; Butterworths.

— and Colcher, A. E. (1937). *Journal of the American Medical Association*, **108**, 867.

— and Forman, M. (1964). Mammography of cancer. *Bulletin of the New York Academy of Medicine*, **40**, 674–689.

— Berger, S. M. and Delpino, L. (1965). Mammography: some remarks on techniques. *Radiologic Clinics of North America*, **3**, 389–401.

— Yiu, L. S. and Berger, S. M. (1962). The diagnostic importance of calcareous patterns in roentgenography of breast cancer. *American Journal of Roentgenology*, **88**, 1117–1125.

Gilbertson, J. D., Randall, M. G. and Fingerhut, A. G. (1970). Evaluation of roentgen exposure in mammography. *Radiology*, **95**, 383–394.

Gravelle, I. H. (1969). Photofluorography. *Odelca Mirror*, **8**, 10–13.

Gros, C. M. (1963). *Les maladies du Sein*. Paris; Masson.

Hicken, N. F. (1937). Mammography. The roentgenographic diagnosis of breast tumours by means of contrast media. *Surgery, Gynecology and Obstetrics*, **64**, 593–603.

Ingleby, H. and Gershon-Cohen, J. (1960). *Comparative Anatomy, Pathology and Roentgenology of the Breast.* Philadelphia; University of Pennsylvania Press.

Kennedy, T. and Biggart, J. D. (1967). Sarcoma of the breast. *British Journal of Cancer*, **21**, 635–644.

Leborgne, R. A. (1953). *The Breast in Roentgen Diagnosis*, Montevideo; Impresora Uraguaya S.A. and London; Constable.

— (1967). Esteatonecrosis quistica calcificada de la mama. *Estudio Radiologico. El Torax*, **16**, 172–175.

— and Dominguez, C. M. (1951). Diagnosis of tumours of the breast by simple roentgenography. *American Journal of Roentgenology*, **65**, 1–11.

Price, J. L. and Butler, P. D. (1970). The reduction of radiation and exposure time in mammography. *British Journal of Radiology*, **43**, 251.

Salomon, A. (1913). Beiträge zur Pathologie and Klinik der Mammacarcinoma. *Archiv fur klinische Chirurgie*, **101**, 573–668.

Samuel, E. and Young, G. B. (1964). *Clinical Surgery*, Vol. I., Chapter 35. Ed. by C. Rob and R. Smith. London; Butterworths.

Sandison, A. T. (1958). Are immediate histological examinations of lumps in the breast useful? *Lancet*, **2**, 338.

Shepherd, T. J., Crile, G. and Strittmatter, W. C. (1962). Roentgenographic evaluation of classifications seen in paraffin block specimens of mammary tumours. *Radiology*, **78**, 967–969.

Stewart, H. J., Gravelle, I. H. and ApSimon, H. T. (1969). Five years' experience with mammography. *British Journal of Surgery*, **56**, 341.

Strax, P., Shapiro, S. and Venet, L. (1968). In *Prognostic Factors in Breast Cancer*, p. 242. Ed. by A. P. M. Forrest and P. B. Kunkler. Edinburgh; Livingstone.

— Venet, L., Shapiro, S. and Gross, S. (1967). *Cancer, Philadelphia*, **20**, 2184.

— — — — and Venet, W. (1969). *Journal of the American Medical Association*, **210**, 433.

Venet, L., Strax, P., Venet, W. and Shapiro, S. (1969). *Cancer, Philadelphia*, **24**, 1187.

Warren, S. L. (1930). Roentgenologic study of breast. *American Journal of Roentgenology*, **24**, 113–124.

— (1940). The relation of "chronic cystic mastitis' to carcinoma of the breast. *Surgery, Gynecology and Obstetrics*, **71**, 257–273.

Wolfe, J. N. (1967a). Mammography: ducts as a sole indicator of breast carcinoma. *Radiology*, **89**, 206–210.

— (1967b). Study of breast parenchyma by mammography in normal women and those with benign and malignant disease. *Radiology*, **89**, 201.

— (1968). Xerography of the breast. *Radiology*, **91**, 231–240.

— (1969a). Xeroradiography of the breast. *Oncology*, **23**, 113–119.

— (1969b). The prominent duct pattern as an indicator of cancer risk. *Oncology*, **23**, 149–158.

Chapter 4

Thermography

HISTORY

Infra-red radiation was so described by Sir William Herschel in 1800. While assessing the heating power of the various colours produced by passing the sun's rays through a prism he noted that maximum heat was produced beyond the visible red of the spectrum. Work on infra-red radiation was continued by his son Sir John, who covered strips of paper with lamp black and then soaked them in alcohol. The alcohol evaporated more rapidly from the portion of the paper exposed to infra-red radiation. These areas appeared lighter in colour producing what he described as a 'thermograph'.

The skin behaves as a black body radiator and constantly emits infra-red radiation in direct proportion to the temperature of its surface. The infra-red waves have a wavelength varying from 4 to 20 µm with a peak emission at 9 µm. Provided a sufficiently sensitive heat detector is available it is possible to measure this radiation at a distance from the patient. The technique of thermography provides a graphic recording of thermal radiation and so it is possible to compare the heat emission of different areas of the body. It is important not to confuse this technique with infra-red photography in which the body is exposed to infra-red radiation and the reflected radiation photographed with an infra-red film.

Lawson in 1957 first showed that in most patients with breast carcinoma the skin over the tumour was warmer than surrounding areas. Subsequent reports by Lloyd Williams *et al.* (1961) and Gershon-Cohen and Haberman in 1964 confirmed these observations.

There is uncertainty as to the origin or nature of the increased heat associated with malignant lesions. Lawson and Gaston (1964) have shown that this heat cannot be entirely vascular since the

103

temperature of the arterial blood supplying the tumour is lower than the venous return. Increased metabolic activity within the tumour is probably responsible for the increased heat. There is evidence that there is some correlation between the degree of temperature rise and the malignancy of the tumour (Williams *et al.*, 1961; Lawson and Chughtai, 1963).

The skin plays a major role in the heat regulating mechanism of the body. It is surrounded by a halo of water vapour. An extensive vascular supply both within and beneath the skin provides a heat exchange system. The calibre of the blood vessels is affected by local stimuli, physical and metabolic factors and by the sympathetic and parasympathetic nervous systems.

There are no heat losses due to sweating at skin temperatures lower than 30°C so, below this, heat loss results from radiation and convection.

APPARATUS AND PRINCIPLES EMPLOYED

There are a number of machines commercially available varying from those with high resolution but slow scanning times to those with instantaneous thermal displays but relatively poor resolution. There has been a marked improvement in the performance of thermographic machines recently and most now have the facility for direct measurement of temperature differences between adjacent parts of the body.

A brief description of the machines currently used is given to indicate the principles on which they are based.

The AGA Thermovision

In this equipment a spherical mirror and oscillating plane mirror focus the incoming infra-red radiation to a rotating prism. The plane mirror oscillates at 16 cycles per second (Hz) and produces a scanning rate of 16 frames per second (f/sec). The prism which rotates at a speed of 200 revolutions per second (rev/sec) transfers the infra-red rays through a secondary lens system to an indium antimonide detector cooled by liquid nitrogen. The amplified electronic signal is displayed on an oscilloscope (*Figure 4.1*) and may be photographed with a Polaroid camera or on panchromatic 35 mm or cine film.

To identify temperature differences in the grey tone picture, isotherms may be produced. An isotherm is a line connecting points of equal temperature and to produce this one temperature along the temperature scale is selected. All points at the selected temperature within the displayed area are then accentuated by increasing the light intensity to saturated white. This manoeuvre produces an 'isotherm'

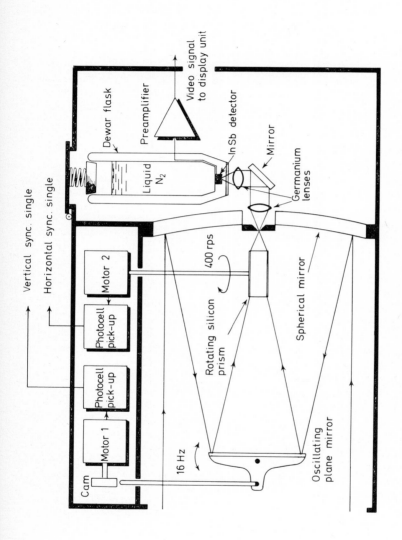

Figure 4.1. Diagrammatic representation of AGA thermovision
(Reproduced by courtesy of AGA (UK) Ltd.)

at the selected temperature. The width of the variable isotherm marker on the grey scale denotes the width of the isotherm temperature. This temperature may be increased or decreased by selected steps by varying the position of the marker on the temperature scale. The isotherms may be photographed and superimposed on the grey tone thermogram or the underlying thermogram may be suppressed leaving the isotherm alone on display. Thus, by means of the isotherm, maps of varying temperature distributions in the breast may be obtained. It is also possible to project the temperature distribution by means of a colour code, each colour representing a different temperature.

The Rank Thermographic System

The camera containing a 10-element detector cooled by liquid nitrogen converts the infra-red radiation to an electronic signal. A high frame rate of 46 per second provides a flicker-free display and a wide scanning angle makes it possible to examine both breasts on one display. The camera has great depth of field and it is possible to compare differences in temperature at selected points along a horizontal display line. This line can be moved vertically anywhere in the display.

The EMI Thermoscan

This scanner allows an easy change from a two-dimensional to a single line scan. The horizontal and vertical fields are scanned by means of rotating plane mirrors. The vertical scanning system can be stopped to give a narrow horizontal line or removed altogether to provide a wide angle scan. The incident energy is focused into a single indium antimonide cell.

It is possible to estimate temperature variations as vertical deflections or as intensity modulation by using a calibrated black level control. In this unit, scanning with highly reflective gold plated mirrors produces a picture with high resolution. It is possible to detect temperature variations as small as $0\cdot1°C$. It has a large field of view corresponding to 2×1 metres at a distance of 5 metres. It is possible to enlarge the central portion of the picture. A 'thermal band' can be inserted in order to interpret thermal variations within the image.

The Pyroscan

The Pyroscan was the first British apparatus to be developed for medical thermography. The detection unit uses an indium antimonide cell cooled with liquid nitrogen. The infra-red radiation is focused by mirrors on to a sensitive indium antimonide cell. A change in conductance in the cell is converted into an equivalent voltage to produce a black and white picture on facsimile paper. Sutherland (1970) has described modifications to the Pyroscan equipping it for temperature profile scanning.

The Barnes Medical Thermograph

This equipment uses a thermistor detector and has a scanning time of about 3 minutes. The thermistor cell needs no cooling and has a wide spectrum of response to infra-red radiation.

TECHNIQUES OF EXAMINATION

Before thermographic examination is carried out the breasts should be cooled in an air conditioned room at an ambient temperature of 19–21°C for 10–15 minutes. The patient's clothing should be removed

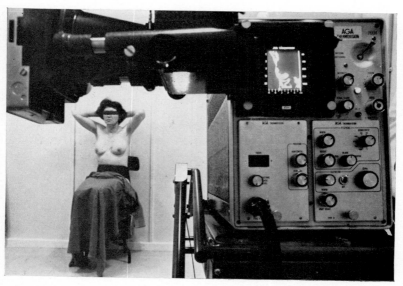

Figure 4.2. Frontal thermography showing position and display on oscilloscope screen

to the waist and the arms raised to allow equal and symmetrical cooling of both breasts. It is possible to hasten cooling of the skin by means of an electric fan or by spraying with alcohol. It is necessary to take frontal and oblique pictures of each breast. Patients can be examined in the supine position provided that the infra-red radiation is reflected into the camera by means of a special highly reflective mirror placed above the patient. This is helpful in those with large pendulous breasts.

The thermograms shown in this Chapter have been produced by the AGA Thermovision equipment. This machine gives a virtually instantaneous picture on a standard oscilloscope. It is possible to connect a slave TV unit to produce a larger picture. The thermal display on the oscilloscope can be photographed either with a Polaroid camera, 35 mm, or cine film. It is possible to identify temperature differences of 0·20°C within a range of $-30°$ to $+200°C$. The minimum focal distance measures 2 metres (*Figure 4.2*).

The oscilloscope provides a grey tone picture and it is possible to choose either a 'white-hot' or 'black-hot' display. Some workers consider that perception is easier with black denoting areas of higher temperature. Additionally, superimposition of an isotherm can indicate areas of identical temperature and also demonstrate areas of increased heat emission. The black-hot display method is used in all the illustrations in this chapter.

The Normal Breast

Thermography provides a pictorial record of the temperature distribution of the breasts. The veins lying subcutaneously are demonstrated as black branching lines due to heat emission. The vascular pattern in a particular patient is constant over a long period of time (Jones and Draper, 1970). There is however marked individual variation in the thermal patterns and few patients have identical venous distributions on each side. The size of the veins also varies from time to time depending partly on the stage of the menstrual cycle.

The axillae are usually hotter than surrounding areas and increased heat emission is often shown at the inferior portion of the breasts, particularly in those with pendulous breasts. In such cases it is often impossible to get adequate cooling in the erect position but this can be achieved more easily in the supine position.

In most normal breasts the nipples are shown to be cool and this contrasts strikingly with the findings in the remainder of the breasts. Variations from this may be seen in some breast carcinomas and infections and also when the nipples are retracted (*Figure 4.3a, b*) or congenitally absent (*Figure 4.3c*). Occasionally neither nipple is shown despite the absence of any clinical evidence of disease. Frequently there is an area of increased heat surrounding the nipple but the nipple itself remains cold (*Figure 4.4*). This is a normal variation and must not be confused with an underlying abnormality. In breast

108

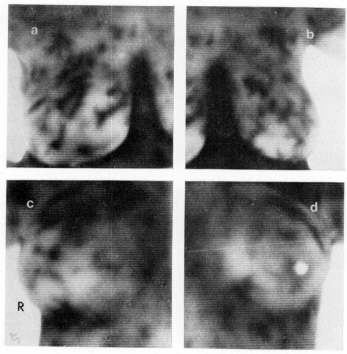

Figure 4.3 (a) and (b). Neither nipple can be identified. There is no clinical abnormality, apart from retraction of the nipples; (c) another patient. Here the right nipple is congenitally absent; (d) normal left breast for comparison

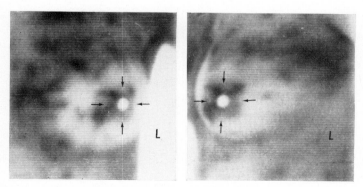

Figure 4.4. 'Halo' around left nipple. This is a normal variation

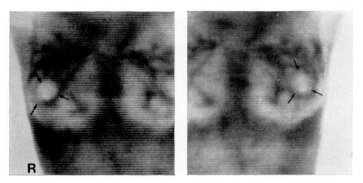

Figure 4.5. The whole of the areola appears cold. This is normal variation

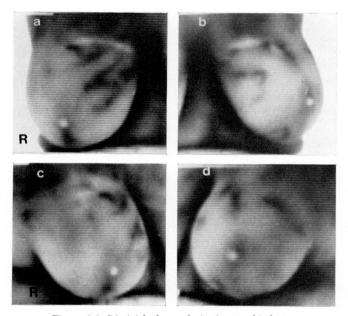

Figure 4.6. Diminished vascularity in atrophic breasts

carcinoma the nipple would be likely to be smaller and hotter than normal though this is not invariable. The whole of the areola may appear cold, particularly in adolescent girls (*Figure 4.5*). In elderly patients with atrophic breasts the vascularity is often diminished compared with that obtaining before the menopause (*Figure 4.6*).

Gross asymmetry of the vascular pattern in post-menopausal women would arouse suspicion of an underlying abnormality in that breast.

INTERPRETATION OF THERMOGRAMS

In thermography of the breast interpretation rests on an assessment of the symmetry or otherwise of the vascular pattern, the appearance of the nipple and the finding of localized or generalized warm areas within the thermographic display. Asymmetrical heat patterns can be due to asymmetry of the superficial venous pattern. Even though this is of no clinical significance it poses a difficult diagnostic problem thermographically as this appearance can be secondary to underlying disease. It is possible to have a temperature difference of up to $1°C$ in normal women but usually temperature differences of more than $1·5°C$ are of significance. However even temperature differences of $4°C$ have been demonstrated in normal women. To add to the difficulty, the left breast is frequently warmer than the right in normal people and often has more numerous veins.

Carcinoma of the Breast

It is important to realize that though dramatic thermographic changes may be shown in carcinoma of the breast the findings are not usually specific and a diagnosis as such cannot be given. Thermography can point to a possible abnormality and on occasions be very important if other investigations are equivocal.

A gross increase in the vascular pattern of the breast in a patient with carcinoma of the breast is a classical finding (*Figures 4.7* and *4.8*). In such cases the thermogram may show that the nipple has remained cold but is smaller than that of the normal breast. Elevation of the nipple may be shown (*Figure 4.9*) and in such cases there is usually increased heat around the nipple and the nipple itself is hotter than that on the opposite side. Of course such a finding would be obvious by clinical examination. In large rapidly growing carcinomas there may be a diffuse increase in the heat emission which obliterates the vascular pattern (*Figures 4.10* and *4.11*).

Less obvious changes associated with a carcinoma include obliteration of the nipple together with a surrounding area of increased heat (*Figure 4.12*) or a solitary enlarged vein overlying a malignant lesion (*Figure 4.13*). Distortion in the outline of the breast may be readily seen (*Figure 4.14*).

111

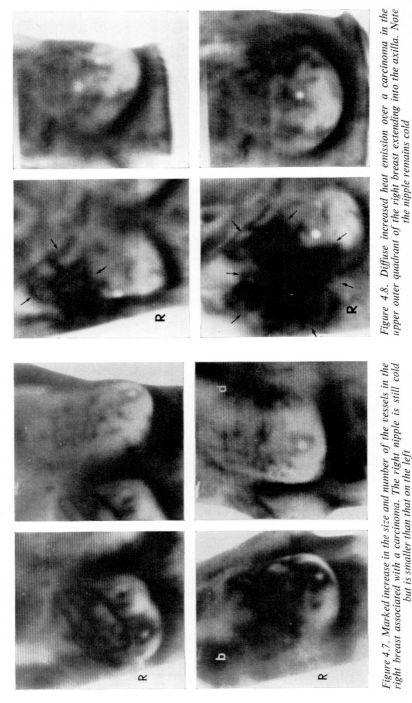

Figure 4.8. Diffuse increased heat emission over a carcinoma in the upper outer quadrant of the right breast extending into the axilla. Note the nipple remains cold

Figure 4.7. Marked increase in the size and number of the vessels in the right breast associated with a carcinoma. The right nipple is still cold but is smaller than that on the left

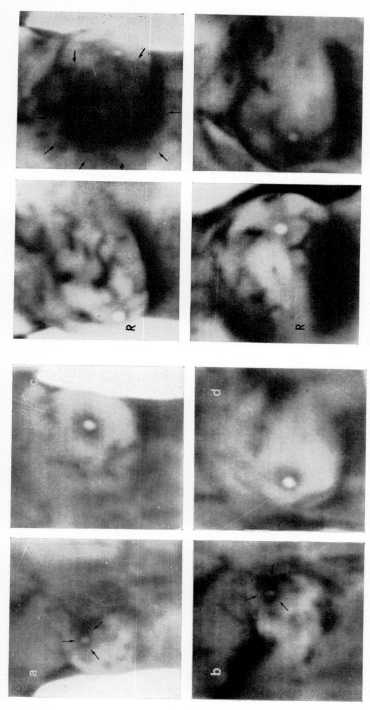

Figure 4.10. Diffuse increased heat over medial aspect of the left breast due to an extensive carcinoma. The vessels on the left side are only slightly increased in size and those in the medial aspect of the breast are obscured

Figure 4.9. Right breast carcinoma showing elevation of the nipple, distortion of the breast and increased heat of the nipple and surrounding area

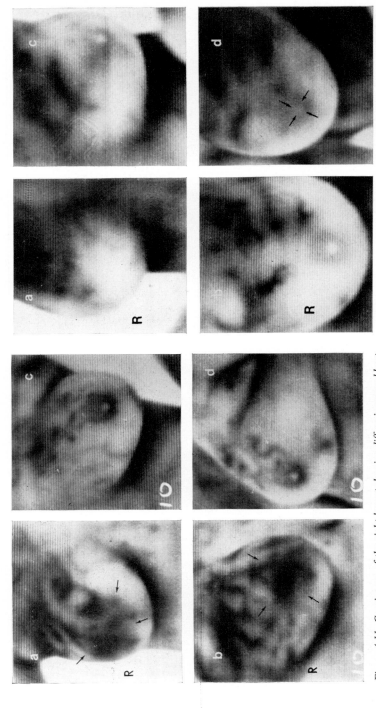

Figure 4.11. Carcinoma of the right breast showing diffuse increased heat emission over the lower outer quadrant of the breast with obliteration of the nipple. The 'halo' around the left nipple is a normal appearance

Figure 4.12. Minimum thermographic changes in carcinoma of the left breast showing 'hot' left nipple

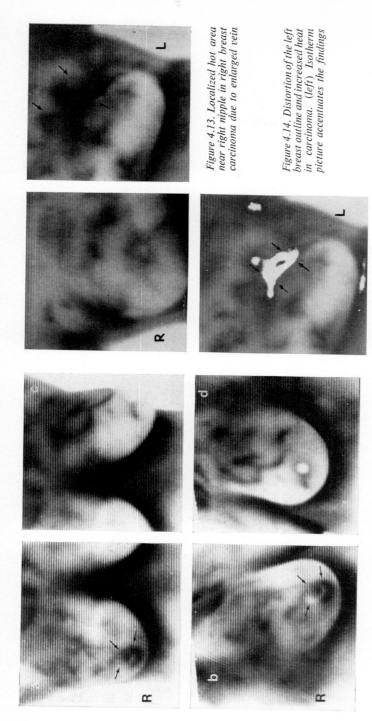

Figure 4.13. Localized hot area near right nipple in right breast carcinoma due to enlarged vein

Figure 4.14. Distortion of the left breast outline and increased heat in carcinoma. (left) Isotherm picture accentuates the findings

Figure 4.14

Figure 4.13

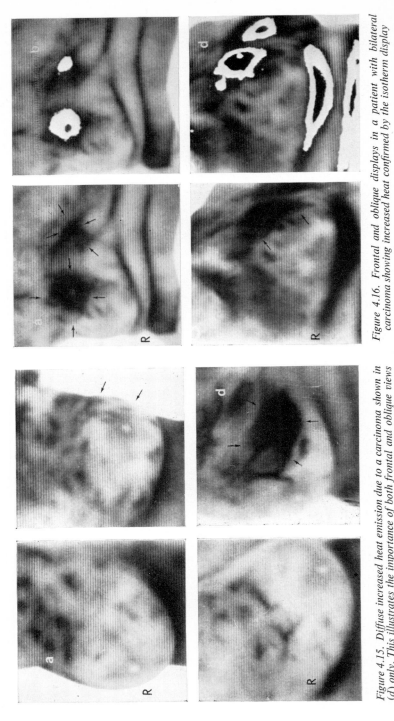

Figure 4.15. Diffuse increased heat emission due to a carcinoma shown in (d) only. This illustrates the importance of both frontal and oblique views

Figure 4.16. Frontal and oblique displays in a patient with bilateral carcinoma showing increased heat confirmed by the isotherm display

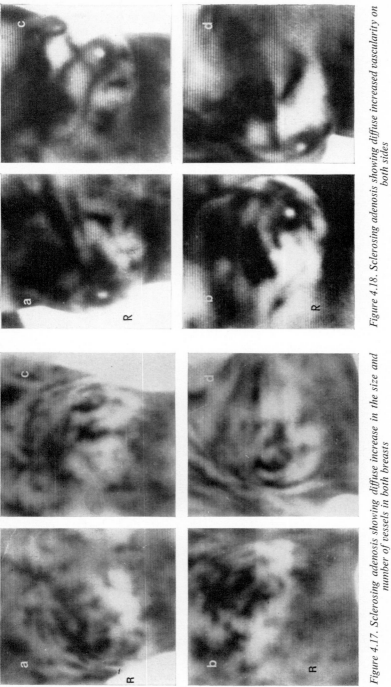

Figure 4.18. Sclerosing adenosis showing diffuse increased vascularity on both sides

Figure 4.17. Sclerosing adenosis showing diffuse increase in the size and number of vessels in both breasts

It is important to take both frontal and oblique views of the breasts because the thermograms may appear completely normal on the frontal view and yet the oblique view may show an abnormality in the lateral half of the breast (*Figure 4.15*). The isotherm is of considerable value, the tumour area showing as saturated white, superimposed on the normal display. The possibility of carcinomas in both breasts should always be considered and in such cases the vascular pattern could be symmetrical and the absence or poor demonstration of the nipples attributed to a normal variation (*Figure 4.16*).

Benign Disease of the Breast

Generalized increase of the size of the vessels may be shown in diffuse disease—e.g., sclerosing adenosis (*Figures 4.17* and *4.18*) or there may be asymmetrical enlargement of the veins indicating an underlying fibroadenoma, cyst or fibroadenosis (*Figure 4.19*). It is

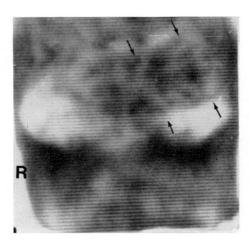

Figure 4.19. Diffuse increased heat over upper part of the left breast. Histology showed fibroadenosis only

important to realize that when there has been previous surgery—e.g., previous removal of a benign lesion of the breast—the area of the scar commonly shows increased heat emission (*Figure 4.20*). The thermographic appearance in such cases may simulate that of malignancy. A cyst of the breast will usually be cold and may show as a well-defined area of diminished heat emission (*Figure 4.21*) but on occasions hypervascularity may be present on the side of the cyst. As would be expected, greatly increased heat emission is present in

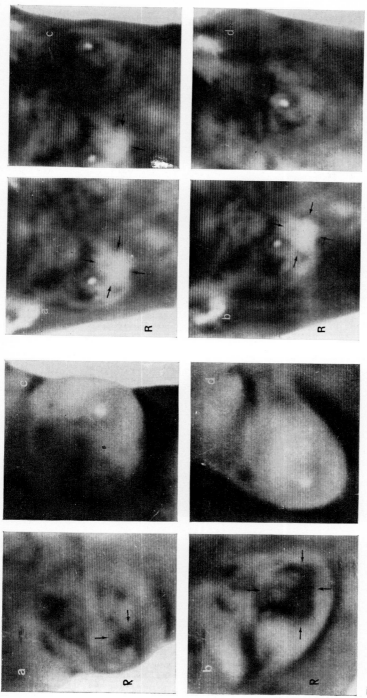

Figure 4.21. Cyst of right breast showing a well-defined 'cold' area corresponding with the position of the cyst

Figure 4.20. Increased heat emission in lower lateral quadrant of the right breast overlying scar following previous removal of fibroadenoma

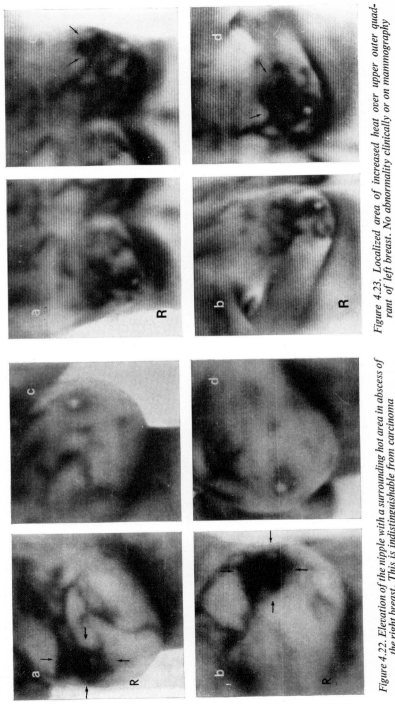

Figure 4.23. Localized area of increased heat over upper outer quadrant of left breast. No abnormality clinically or on mammography

Figure 4.22. Elevation of the nipple with a surrounding hot area in abscess of the right breast. This is indistinguishable from carcinoma

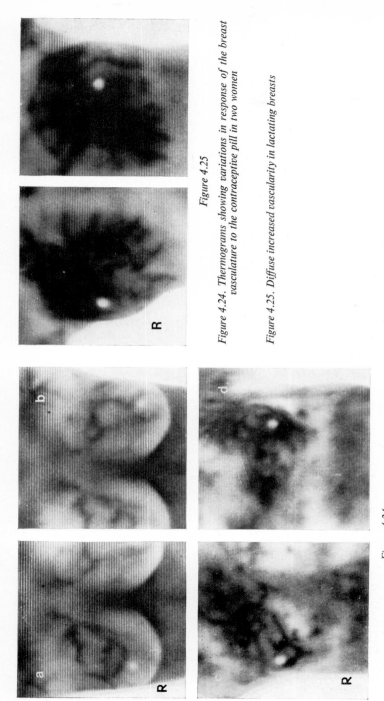

Figure 4.25

Figure 4.24. Thermograms showing variations in response of the breast vasculature to the contraceptive pill in two women

Figure 4.25. Diffuse increased vascularity in lactating breasts

Figure 4.24

patients with breast abscesses, the appearances being identical with those found in breast carcinoma (*Figure 4.22*). A repeat examination after a short course of antibiotics may help to solve this particular problem.

Abnormal Thermograms in Apparently Normal Breasts

A great problem arises when an abnormal thermal pattern is produced in patients without clinical evidence of breast disease (*Figure 4.23*). Asymmetry of the vascular pattern can be normal and care should be taken not to produce needless anxiety in such cases. If there is doubt following clinical examination and mammography in such cases then biopsy should be undertaken. If however the clinical and mammographic examinations are normal then serial thermographic and clinical examinations are a wise policy.

Physiological Changes in the Breast

In pregnancy the thermographic pattern of the breasts shows increased vascularity and this can sometimes be seen as early as 2 weeks after conception (Birnbaum, 1966). Likewise, oral contraceptives can sometimes give a similar appearance although this is not inevitable. For these reasons interpretation of breast disease by thermography is rendered somewhat more difficult (*Figure 4.24*). As one would expect during lactation, there is a great increase in the heat emission and the vessels within the breasts become larger (*Figure 4.25*). Diurnal variation of temperature may be noted (Samuel, 1968).

Isard and Shilo (1968) attempted to correlate the phase of the menstrual cycle with the appearances on thermography. It seemed that in some patients there was increased vascularity of the breast one week before the menstrual period whereas repeat studies one week later showed diminution in vascularity. This however only occurred in half of the cases and there is consequently no accurate correlation between the thermographic pattern and the phase of the menstrual cycle. The authors concluded that this finding seems to be of no particular significance in the management of breast lesions.

EVALUATION

There is considerable difference of opinion regarding the accuracy of thermography in the detection of breast carcinoma. Characteristic thermographic patterns include a diffuse increase in heat emission on the affected side, increased vascularity, a hot nipple and local or generalized hot areas. Unfortunately, thermography may be completely normal in clinically evident breast carcinomas (*Figure 4.26*)

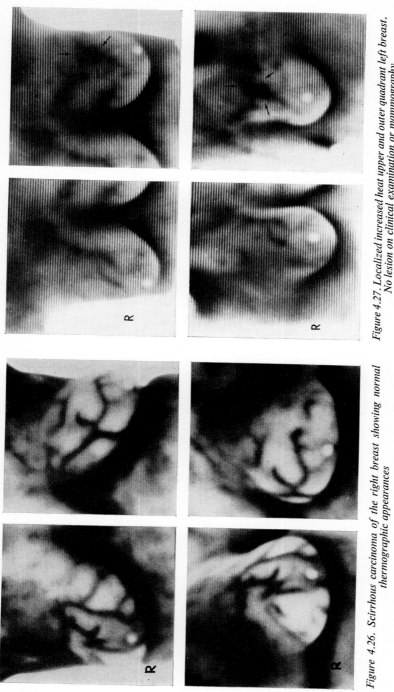

Figure 4.27. Localized increased heat upper and outer quadrant left breast. No lesion on clinical examination or mammography

Figure 4.26. Scirrhous carcinoma of the right breast showing normal thermographic appearances

whereas appearances simulating breast carcinoma may be present in patients without clinical or mammographic evidence of disease (*Figures 4.23* and *4.27*). On one occasion in our series a carcinoma was diagnosed thermographically in the right breast whereas it was actually present in the left breast (*Figure 4.28*). Isard, Ostrum and Shilo (1969) found that in 76 malignant lesions the thermograms

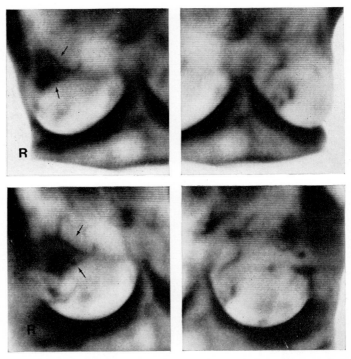

Figure 4.28. Increased heat upper outer quadrant right breast diagnosed as a carcinoma. A carcinoma was however present in the left breast. This cannot be identified

were positive in 72 per cent whereas in the benign group 61 per cent of the thermograms were positive. They stated that they were unable to differentiate the benign from the malignant patterns by thermography. On the other hand, Swearingen (1965) found that in none of the 86 patients in his series with malignant tumours proved by biopsy was a thermogram negative. He commented, however, that there were many false positive diagnoses but these showed a return to normal after an interval. Gershon-Cohen *et al.* (1970) reported 4 patients with breast cancer who came to biopsy as a result of elevated skin temperatures as shown by thermography.

A report on the use of thermography on 2,523 volunteer women who were screened for breast cancer has been published by Hitchcock *et al.* (1968). They found that there was an unacceptably large group in whom the thermogram was abnormal but no subsequent lesion was found. Out of 4 patients diagnosed as having breast carcinoma only 1 was found by thermography.

Similar findings were reported by Nathan *et al.* (1970) who analysed the thermographic findings in 97 patients referred to their breast clinic. Out of 16 patients with breast carcinoma 4 were normal thermographically. Furthermore, a large number of false positives were found. Furnival *et al.* (1970) compared the value of clinical examination, thermography and 70 mm photofluorography in 416 patients presenting with symptoms of breast disease and 417 asymptomatic volunteers. The mammograms and thermograms were interpreted independently by three radiologists who had no knowledge of the findings on clinical examination. There was wide inter-observer variation, but taking the best of three observers in only 51·9 per cent of 77 patients with breast carcinoma was the diagnosis suggested by thermography. All three observers wrongly diagnosed 32·5 per cent of these cases. In 3 patients however, thermography had suggested the diagnosis of carcinoma when clinical examination and mammography had indicated benign lesions. Undoubtedly the accuracy of thermography would have been improved if access to clinical findings had been made available.

Thermography was used as part of a screening programme for breast cancer from a 'well woman' clinic by Davey *et al.* (1970). Of 1,717 thermograms, 197 showed abnormal heat patterns, and of 15 malignant cases, 11 had positive thermographic findings. Some of those with abnormal heat patterns were subjected to re-examination clinically and had mammography performed. Two further carcinomas were found by this method.

Price (1970) compared mammography and thermography in 150 patients with breast symptoms. In 28 patients with breast carcinoma 5 were normal thermographically. Three patients with breast carcinoma had equivocal findings clinically and suspicious mammograms but positive thermograms. False positive thermograms were found in 5 patients. He concluded that though thermography is a valuable adjunct to mammography, women with breast carcinoma can on occasion be given false reassurance and those with a false positive diagnosis suffer needless anxiety.

Stark and Way (1970) showed that the introduction of thermography as a method additional to palpation improved the detection rate for breast carcinoma but 6 patients subsequently shown to have breast cancer were initially considered negative. However they considered that an unacceptable number of patients with breast carcinoma was missed by these methods. One large carcinoma showed normal thermographic appearances. However a combination of palpation, thermography and mammography has proved satisfactory as in 850 high risk women, 13 were found to have early breast cancer.

Thermography was further evaluated by Nathan *et al.* (1972) who reported their experience of this technique in the differential diagnosis of 359 patients most of whom had presented with breast symptoms. In 195 of these the breast thermogram was interpreted as abnormal but 115 of these patients had no clinical evidence of disease, a false positive incidence of 59 per cent. Of 164 patients with normal thermograms, 41 had benign lesions and 7 had breast cancer giving a false negative incidence of 29 per cent.

In a 'well woman' clinic, Davey *et al.* (1972) reported that 15 patients with breast carcinoma were discovered in the first 2,700 patients. Only 8 of these had a palpable lesion but 10 had positive thermograms.

It is therefore clear that there is a considerable difference of opinion between observers as to the value of thermography in breast disease. Most workers agree that differentiation between benign and malignant lesions is often impossible. The technique is useful, however, because it can detect an area of increased heat emission suggesting an underlying abnormality. It has been emphasized that apparently normal patients may have abnormal thermograms and those with carcinoma may give normal results. Nonetheless, while these deficiencies of the technique are appreciated, thermography has a part to play. In survey work the thermogram can give additional supporting evidence to clinical or mammographic findings. We do not believe that thermography should be used as an isolated examination because it is not sufficiently accurate and it can produce unnecessary anxiety by giving a false positive result. Furthermore it may give a false feeling of security to some patients with breast carcinoma.

It is possible that patients with false positive results—i.e., abnormal thermograms—may be at high risk of subsequently developing breast cancer. This will only become evident when persons with such findings are followed up for an extended period. An alteration in the thermographic picture may be of considerable diagnostic importance in such patients.

REFERENCES

Thermography

Birnbaum, S. J. (1966). Breast temperature as a test for pregnancy. *Obstetrics and Gynecology, New York*, **27**, 378–380.

Connell, J. F., Ruzicka, F. F., Grossi, C. E., Osborne, A. W. and Conte, A. J. (1966). Thermography in the detection of breast cancer. *Cancer, Philadelphia*, **19**, 83–88.

Davey, Jane B., Greening, W. P. and McKinna, J. A. (1970). Is screening for cancer worth while? Results from a well-woman clinic for cancer detection. *British Medical Journal*, **3**, 696–699.

— Richter, Annabel and Pentney, B. H. (1972). Correspondence on 'value of thermography'. *British Medical Journal*, **2**, 590.

Draper, J. W. and Jones, C. H. (1969). Thermal patterns of the female breast. *British Journal of Radiology*, **42**, 401–410.

Gershon-Cohen, J. and Haberman, J. D. (1964). Thermography. *Radiology*, **82**, 280–285.

— Hermel, M. B. and Murdock, M. G. (1970). Thermography in detection of early breast cancer. *Cancer, Philadelphia*, **26**, 1153–1156.

Hitchcock, C. R., Hickok, D. F., Soucheray, J., Moulton, T. and Baker, R. C. (1968). Thermography in mass screening for occult breast cancer. *Journal of the American Medical Association*, **204**, 419–422.

Isard, H. J. and Shilo, R. (1968). Breast thermography. *The American Journal of Roentgenology, Radium Therapy and Nuclear Medicine*, **103**, 921–925.

— Ostrum, B. J. and Shilo, R. (1969). Thermography in breast carcinoma. *Surgery, Gynecology and Obstetrics*, **128**, 1289–1292.

Jones, C. H. and Draper, J. W. (1970). A comparison of infrared photography and thermography in the detection of mammary carcinoma. *British Journal of Radiology*, **43**, 507–516.

Lawson, R. N. (1957). Thermography: A new tool in investigation of breast lesions. *Canadian Services Medical Journal*, **13**, 517–524.

— and Chughtai, M. S. (1963). Breast cancer and body temperature. *Canadian Medical Association Journal*, **88**, 68–70.

— and Gaston, J. P. (1964). Temperature measurements of localised pathological processes. *Annals of the New York Academy of Sciences*, **121**, 90–98.

Lloyd Williams, K., Lloyd Williams, F. and Handley, R. S. (1960). Infra-red radiation thermometry in clinical practice. *Lancet*, **2**, 958–959.

— — — (1961). Infra-red thermometry in the diagnosis of breast disease. *Lancet*, **2**, 1378–1381.

Nathan, B. E., Galasko, C. S. B. and Pallett, J. E. (1970). Thermography in breast cancer. *British Journal of Surgery*, **57**, 518–520.

— Ian Burn, J. and MacErlean, D. P. (1972). Value of mammary thermography in differential diagnosis. *British Medical Journal*, **2**, 316–317.

Parry, C. E. Freundlich, I. W. and Wallace, A. B. (1972). Breast thermograms in ovulatory and anovulatory menstrual cycles. *British Journal of Radiology*, **45**, 507–509.

127

Price, J. L. (1970). Screening for breast cancer. *Lancet*, **2**, 927.

Samuel, E. (1968). Medical aspects of thermography. *British Journal of Hospital Medicine*, Equipment Supplement, 8.

Stark, A. M. and Way, S. (1970). Screening for breast cancer. *Lancet*, **2**, 407–409.

Sutherland, W. H. (1970). Temperature profile scanning—a more quantitative approach to thermography. *Bio-Medical Engineering*, **5**, 493–500.

Swearingen, A. G. (1965). Thermography: report of the radiographic and thermographic examinations of the breasts of 100 patients. *Radiology*, **85**, 818–824.

Chapter 5

Ultrasonography

HISTORY

Ultrasonic techniques have been developed for examination of the breast and reports have already been published. Wild (1950) showed how ultrasound could be used to measure thickness of tissues and detect changes in tissue density. In 1952, Wild and Reid published the first two-dimensional ultrasonic scans of the breast. In 1954, Howry, Stott and Bliss satisfactorily demonstrated carcinoma of the breast and in 1962 Hayashi *et al.* showed how breast carcinoma could be diagnosed by means of a linear scanner. Again, using a linear scanner, Evans *et al.* (1966) were able to demonstrate breast cysts.

Ultrasonic breast scanning may be carried out either by placing the probe in direct contact with the skin or by immersing the breasts in water, the probe being at a distance from the skin surface. Technically, it is difficult to carry out efficient contact scanning of the breasts. There are no commercial machines available to carry out indirect scanning using a water bath. Wagai *et al.* (1972) have described an immersion method in which ultrasonic pulsed waves are transmitted through a vinyl bag full of degassed water. The ultrasonic examinations demonstrated in this section have been performed with an instrument designed solely for this purpose. In this machine the breasts are suspended in water and a B-scope display system is used (Wells and Evans, 1968).

TECHNIQUES OF EXAMINATION

The majority of ultrasonic techniques employ a system of reflection rather than one of direct transmission as used in radiography. When the ultrasonic beam encounters an interface such as the skin surface

129

a proportion of the ultrasound is reflected back to the transmitter which then acts as a receiver. The echo obtained is recorded on a cathode ray oscilloscope as a dot of light at a point which represents spatially the position of the echo-producing interface within the body. Summation of the echoes produces a cross-sectional picture on the oscilloscope which can be recorded on Polaroid or 35 mm film.

The patient lies prone on a fibre glass couch above a water-filled tank enclosing the scanning system (*Figure 5.1a*). The breasts project through a rectangular hole in the couch so that they are immersed in water which is at a constant temperature of 37°C. The water is kept sterile by the addition of Savlon Concentrate and the tank is emptied and re-filled at regular intervals. The upright console contains the receiver/amplifier system, the transmitter with output control, the display oscilloscope and a camera.

During the scan the ultrasonic probe passes horizontally beneath the patient. At the same time it rotates on an angle of 38 degrees. This rocking movement ensures that the ultrasonic beam enters the patient from many different angles. An echo can be recorded from an interface within the breast only if the interface is at right-angles to the ultra-sonic beam. The system is illustrated diagrammatically in *Figure 5.1b*.

A scan is first obtained through the thickest portion of both breasts. This is recorded with a Polaroid camera and viewed immediately. It is necessary to ensure that the breasts have been sufficiently penetrated by ultrasound. If this scan appears satisfactory subsequent scans are recorded on 35 mm panchromatic film. This has the advantage of cheapness and improved detail compared with Polaroid film. Scans are taken at intervals of 1 cm from the superior to the inferior aspects of both breasts so that multiple cross-sectional displays of the breasts can be obtained. A single scan of both breasts can be achieved in 16 seconds. The scans are viewed on a Hansen viewer in order to magnify the images.

The complex internal structure of the breast, varying from patient to patient, makes diagnosis by ultrasound difficult. Each ultrasonic scan contains a cross-sectional display of both breasts so it is possible to compare the appearances on each side. When examining the scans it is necessary to note whether or not skin thickening is present or whether there is a relative increase or decrease in the number of echoes.

Each scan shows the skin surface, the skin itself appearing as a rela-tively thick white line. Beneath the skin a relatively transonic area is generally present due to the subcutaneous fat. The glandular tissue of the breast reflects ultrasound and will consequently be represented

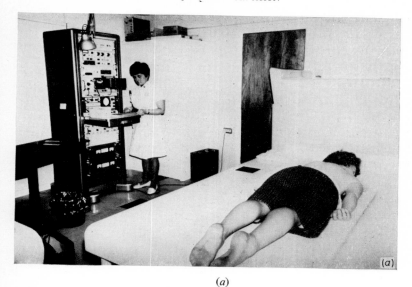

(a)

Horizontal section   Longitudinal section

Water   bath

(b)

Figure 5.1. (a) Ultrasonic breast scanner; (b) diagrammatic cross-section illustrating principle

by a collection of echoes varying in size according to the relative amounts of glandular and fatty tissue. Because an interface between tissue and air or gas reflects ultrasound almost completely the chest wall is clearly delineated on each scan.

In general terms solid lesions within the breast will reflect more ultrasound in comparison with the surrounding normal breast or the opposite breast. In some cases the lesion may be impenetrable by ultrasound, producing an echo-free zone beyond. Fluid-containing lesions allow the ultrasonic beam to pass through unhindered so that the posterior aspect of such lesions is clearly seen and the lesions themselves appear transonic.

INTERPRETATION IN ULTRASONOGRAPHY

Carcinoma of the Breast

Because a solid lesion within the breast will reflect ultrasound an increased number of echoes may be seen at the site of the tumour. It is particularly important to compare the relatively transonic subcutaneous regions on both sides. An increased number of echoes strongly suggests malignant infiltration (*Figure 5.2*). Comparison with other methods of examination will assist in making the correct diagnosis (*Figures 5.3, 5.4* and *5.6*). On occasions the whole breast may show increased echoes with virtual obliteration of the subcutaneous space (*Figure 5.3a*). The extent of a lesion may not readily be shown—particularly if the ultrasonic beam is so attenuated by the surface of the tumour that an echo-free zone beyond it appears. The true nature of the lesion can be assessed by comparison with mammograms (*Figure 5.4*). Extensive skin thickening may be evident (*Figure 5.5*). A mucoid carcinoma may appear transonic because there is less attenuation of the beam due to the semi-fluid nature of the tumour (*Figure 5.6*).

Benign Breast Disease

It is not possible at present by ultrasonic methods to identify diffuse bilateral benign breast disease. Fibroadenomas may be shown if they are over 1 cm in size. In such cases it is necessary to scan the breasts completely at 1 cm intervals because large distances between sections could result in the ultrasonic beam missing a small lesion. Small solid tumours may produce a cluster of echoes (*Figure 5.7*) and in such cases it may be very difficult to differentiate ultrasonically between a fibroadenoma and a carcinoma.

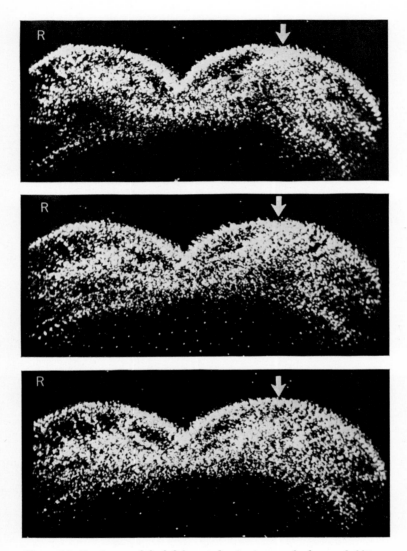

Figure 5.2. Carcinoma of the left breast showing increased echoes and oblitera-tion of the normal transonic fat lines

133

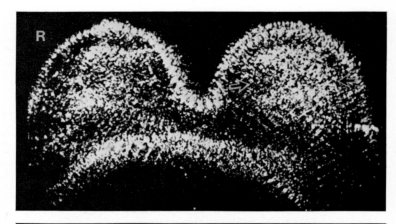

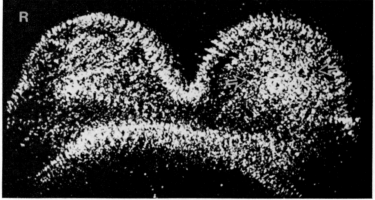

Figure 5.3. (a) Consecutive ultrasonic tomograms showing increased echoes on the left side due to an extensive carcinoma

Cysts of the breast are readily identifiable. A completely transonic area within the breast is characteristic of this lesion (*Figure 5.8*). Many of these cysts are lax and not easily palpated. Both ultrasound and mammography may show such lesions (*Figure 5.9*).

EVALUATION

Ultrasound produces mechanical vibrations which do not cause the kind of damage attributed to x-rays. In the frequency range and intensity used in diagnosis, no clinical or experimental evidence of

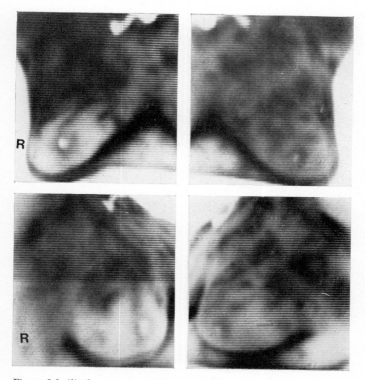

Figure 5.3. (b) thermograms in the same patient showing diffuse increase in heat emission from the left breast

harmful effects has been shown. The examination is painless and can be repeated as often as necessary. With the apparatus at present available the resolution is such that its value as a diagnostic tool is somewhat limited. On occasions it is impossible to differentiate between a carcinoma and surrounding breast tissue. Its value at the moment lies in the ease of differentiating a cystic from a solid lesion.

Particularly encouraging results have been reported by Wagai *et al.* (1972) in the investigation of Japanese patients with breast carcinoma. Their diagnostic accuracy of breast carcinoma was 90·2 per cent with a false positive incidence in benign disease of 11·9 per cent. The minimum size of a lesion diagnosed by ultrasound was 0·7 cm in diameter. They emphasized that ultrasound is more effective than mammography for the diagnosis of cystic lesions.

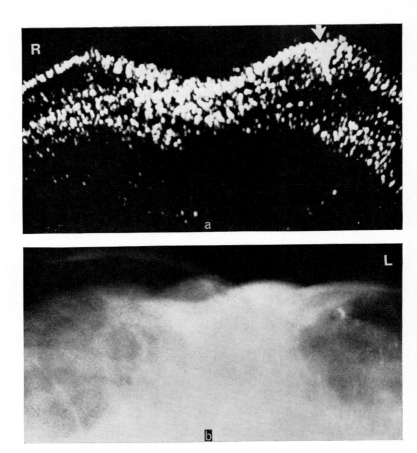

Figure 5.4. (a) Ultrasonogram showing triangular collection of echoes behind left nipple due to carcinoma. An echo-free zone beyond results from attenuation of the beam from absorption within the tumour. There is localized skin thickening also; (b) mammogram of same patient showing retraction of nipple and evidence of a mass with malignant calcification and skin thickening in the left breast

With further technical development of apparatus, ultrasonography may provide yet another method to be used routinely in the search for early breast carcinoma.

SUMMARY

Mammography is a well established ancillary method of examination in breast disease. It is of proved value and high degrees of diagnostic accuracy may be achieved by this means. Definitive diagnoses may be made as detailed demonstration of normal breast structures and abnormal lesions is to be expected. Impalpable carcinoma may readily be demonstrated and accurately localized.

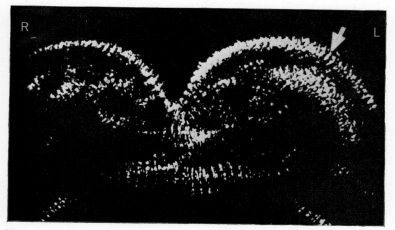

Figure 5.5. Extensive skin thickening with underlying carcinoma showing increased echo pattern

Reproduced from Wells (1969), by courtesy of the author and Academic Press.)

The great disadvantage of thermography in examination of the breast is its non-specificity. The signs of malignant disease are similar to those of benign disease and at times to normal breast variants. The thermogram may show an abnormal vascular and heat pattern but it is not usually possible to diagnose the exact nature of the underlying breast lesion from the thermographic abnormality alone. However, very occasionally a thermographic abnormality may be the only abnormal finding in occult carcinoma of the breast. Thermographic examination may also be of help in evaluating equivocal mammographic findings.

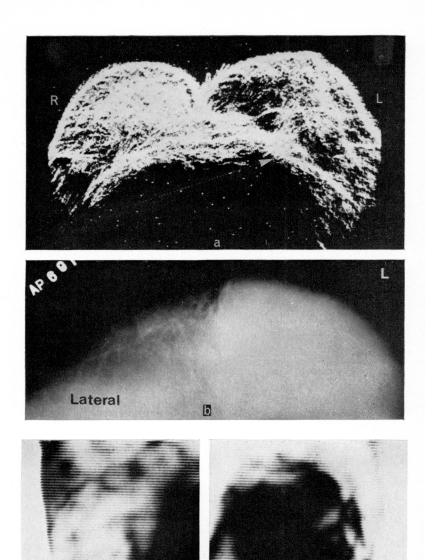

Figure 5.6. Mucoid carcinoma: (a) the transonic nature of the tumour is shown in the medial half of the left breast; (b) mammogram showing the circumscribed nature of the tumour; (c) extensive hypervascularity and increased heat emission over the tumour

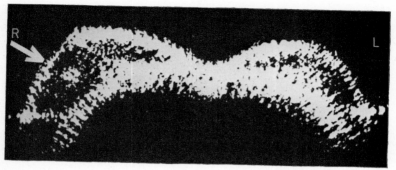

Figure 5.7. Small group of echoes in right breast due to a fibroadenoma
(Reproduced from Wells (1969), by courtesy of the author and Academic Press.)

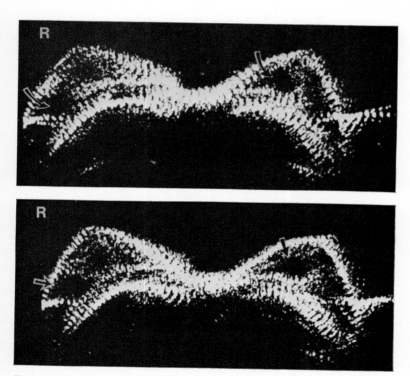

Figure 5.8. Rounded transonic areas in both breasts indicating cysts. The cyst on the left side only was palpable

139

As yet, little attention has been paid to ultrasound as a means of investigating breast disease. It certainly provides a simple and accurate method of distinguishing between cystic and solid lesions. Differentiation of benign and malignant disease is also possible but,

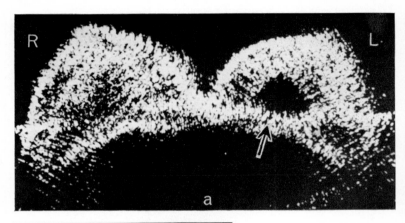

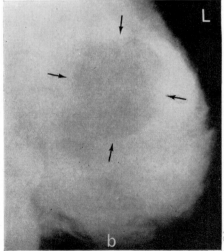

Figure 5.9. (a) Ultrasonogram showing transonic area in left breast due to a cyst; (b) mammogram after aspiration of cyst and replacement with air

((*a*) Reproduced from Wells (1969), by courtesy of the author and Academic Press.)

as already stressed, the resolving power of the available apparatus is limited at present. However, technical developments may allow more detailed examination in the future and so open up another dimension in the examination of the breast.

140

REFERENCES

Ultrasound

Evans, G. C., Lehman, J. S., Brady, L. W., Smyth, M. G. and Hart, D. J. (1966). 'Ultrasonic scanning of abdominal and pelvic organs using the B-scan display.' In *Diagnostic Ultrasound*, pp. 369–415. Ed. by C. C. Grossman, J. H. Holmes, C. Joyner and E. W. Purnell. New York; Plenum Press.

Hayashi, S., Wagai, T., Miyazawa, R., Ito, K., Ishikawa, S., Uematsu, K., Kikuchi, Y. and Uchida, R. (1962). Ultrasonic diagnosis of breast tumour and cholelithiasis. *Western Journal of Surgery, Obstetrics and Gynecology*, **70**, 34–40.

Howry, D. H., Stott, D. A. and Bliss, W. R. (1954). Ultrasonic visualisation of carcinoma of breast and other soft tissue structures. *Cancer, New York*, **7**, 354–358.

Wagai, T., Tsutsumi, M., Ishihara, A., Hadidi, A. M. and Hayashi, S. (1972). Detection of the breast cancer at an early stage by ultrasonic scanning method. Annual Report of The Medical Ultrasonics Research Centre. Japan; Juntendo University School of Medicine.

Wells, P. N. (1969). *Physical principles of Ultrasonic Diagnosis*, Vol. I, Ch. 4, p. 167. New York; Academic Press.

— and Evans, K. T. (1968). An immersion scanner for two dimensional ultrasonic examination of the human breast. *Ultrasonics*, **6**, 220.

Wild, J. J. (1950). The use of ultrasonic pulses for the measurement of biologic tissues and the detection of tissue density change. *Surgery, St. Louis*, **27**, 183–188.

— and Reid, J. M. (1952a). Application of echo-ranging techniques to the determination of structure of biological tissues. *Science, New York*, **115**, 226–230.

— — (1952b). Future pilot echographic studies on the histologic structure of the living intact human breast. *American Journal of Pathology*, **28**, 839–861.

— — (1954). Echographic visualisation of lesions of the living intact human breast. *Cancer Research*, **14**, 277–283.

Index

Traumatic lesions, 31
  fat necrosis following, 39
Tuberculous cold abscess, 36
Tuberculous mastitis, 72

Ultrasonography, 129–141
  accuracy, 135
  benign disease, in, 132, 134
  carcinoma, in, 129, 132–134, 136–
    138
  evaluation of, 134
  history, 129
  interpretation, 132
  technique, 129–132

Vascular appearances, 26, 27
  adenosis, in, 39
  carcinoma, in, 69, 72
  chronic abscess, in, 38
  giant fibroadenoma, in, 33, 35
  infection, in, 72
  lobular carcinoma, in, 52
Veins
  engorgement
    abscess, in, 63
    adenosis, in, 62
  enlargement of, 26

Xeroradiography, 13, 14